# WHY WON'T MY MEDICATION WORK?

## William Edward Ackerman III, MD

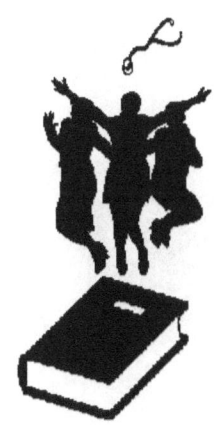

WHY WON'T MY MEDICATION WORK?

Copyright © 2015 by William Edward Ackerman III, MD

All rights reserved. No part of this book may be reproduced or transmitted in any form or by any means without written permission of the author.

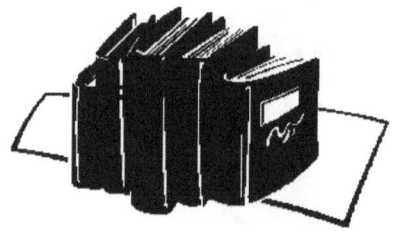

This book is dedicated to my significant other whom I love and cherish.

# Acknowledgments

I wish to acknowledge my patients. Their questions that they asked concerning their medications and why their medications work or do not work prompted the writing of this book. If a patient has a basic understanding of their pathology and what their medication is supposed to do, and why it doesn't work, it helps he or she cope better with their with frustration with their treatment and helps the treating physician better understand his or her patient concerns and ultimately provide better care.

# Foreword

When you take a medication, you expect it to give you benefit. For example, if you have a headache, you would want to take a headache medication, and you would expect then to have relief of your headache. Most individuals realize that this does not always happen. Not every medication works for everyone who takes it, and this it is completely normal. A medication that works for your neighbor may not work for you. The purpose of this book is to provide you with some insight as to why medicines do not always work. New drugs and other modalities are being introduced with increasing frequency. A patient needs to partner with his or her doctor and become involved in their pharmacologic treatment. The reason for this book is to give a patient the basic information necessary to rationally discuss his or her medication failure with the treating physician.

## Table of Contents

1. Pharmacology Basics ............................................................. 1
2. Drug Metabolism ................................................................. 11
3. Drug Interactions ................................................................ 15
4. Gender Factor ..................................................................... 21
5. Generic or Brand Name? ..................................................... 29
7. How Drugs are made .......................................................... 39
8. Herbal "Drugs" ................................................................... 47
9. Drug Laws in the United States .......................................... 53
10. Drug Abuse ....................................................................... 57
11. Drug Dosing ...................................................................... 65
12. Drug Effects in the Elderly ................................................ 75
13. Drugs in Pediatric Patients ................................................ 81
14. Drug Reactions .................................................................. 89
15. Genetic Testing .................................................................. 95
16. Anti-Inflammatory Drugs ................................................. 103
17. Pain Medications .............................................................. 119
18. Local Anesthetics .............................................................. 135
19. Neuropharmacology .......................................................... 145
20. Psychopharmacology ........................................................ 159
21. Hypertensive Drugs .......................................................... 173
22. Gastrointestinal Drugs ...................................................... 183
23. Diabetes and Thyroid Drugs ............................................. 191

24. Chemotherapy ................................................................. 203
25. Antibiotic and Antiviral Medications............................ 217
26. Hormones ..................................................................... 235
27. Erectile Dysfunction Drugs.......................................... 245
28. Muscle Relaxants ......................................................... 253
29. Sleep Medications ........................................................ 265
30. Laxatives ...................................................................... 275
31. Autoimmune drugs....................................................... 283
32. Birth Control Pills ....................................................... 291
33. Cardiac Drugs .............................................................. 297
34. Pulmonary Drugs ......................................................... 309
35. Blood Thinners............................................................. 315

# 1. Pharmacology Basics

A medication is a drug used to treat an illness. The drug that you take goes from outside your body to a specific area in your body called a target receptor. This is the area on your body here your medication is supposed to work (heart, lung, etc.). This drug-receptor action is dependent on your specific pharmacodynamics and kinetics. Pharmacodynamics is the science of how a drug works for your body. This is called the mechanism of action of the drug which determines how a drug gives you pain relief. Pharmacokinetics, on the other hand, is the study of how drugs enter your body; reach their site of action (your heart, brain, etc.), and how they are eliminated from your body. Drug absorption is a drug's progress from the time it's administered until it reaches your blood systemic circulation.

There are two major types of drug actions: 1. Drugs which change your body cells from within the cell (e.g. an antacid can stop acid production in some stomach cells). 2. Another drug action is where drugs bind to receptors on the outside of your cells and change your cell's function. For example, a drug-receptor interaction (Lock and Key Mechanism) may occur when a drug attaches to your cell receptors. Think of receptors on the outside of your pain transmitting cells in your spinal cord and brain as doors. If you close and lock the doors with a medication, you won't let pain signals get to your brain's pain processing cells, which decrease pain perception.

Morphine can lock a receptor and keep the cell from receiving pain signals. As a result, your pain will be decreased. An agonist is a chemical which binds to a specific receptor on a cell and produces an effect by stimulating the receptor such as a nerve pain cell which ultimately can cause your pain. An example is Substance P, which stimulates nerve cells to transmit pain signals to your brain and spinal cord. This chemical unlocks and opens the doors on your cells and therefore, permits pain signals to travel from door to door until they reach your brain. The goal in pain management is to use the correct drug to lock the doors so that you will stop hurting. On the other hand, an antagonist is a drug which binds to a specific receptor and blocks other substances from stimulating the receptor. Morphine, for example, binds with a receptor and stops the nerve cell from transmitting pain signals to your brain.

There are some important terms for you to know. Affinity is the ability of a drug to bind to its receptor (like a magnet to a refrigerator). Efficacy is the ability of a drug to stimulate a receptor. Competitive inhibition occurs when an agonist and antagonist compete for occupation at the same receptor site. Morphine (agonist) and Narcan (antagonist) may compete for the same receptor on a cell. Narcan can antagonize the pain relieving effects of morphine by removing the morphine molecule (the key) from the door (your cell receptor).

Most drugs need to be absorbed from your stomach or small intestine in order to get to the receptors where they are designed to go. Drug absorption describes how drugs enter your bloodstream. The different methods of drug administration are: (1) oral and sublingual. Approximately 80% of drugs used in medical practice are given orally. This route is convenient and economical. A certain drug is ingested and absorbed from your stomach or your intestine. The drug subsequently enters your circulation and goes to your liver where metabolism begins and then enters your blood stream.

A drug can be dissolved under your tongue and is then absorbed through mucous membranes in your mouth into your bloodstream. An example is nitroglycerin sublingual tablets. Transdermal is where a drug is contained in a patch and is absorbed through your skin. An advantage of this route is that the drug dosage is continuous and long-acting. An example is the fentanyl patch. Rectal administration is where the drug is in a suppository form and is inserted through the rectum and is absorbed from the bloodstream. This route may be used for unconscious or vomiting patients. Inhalation administration is when the drug is inhaled through your lungs as a gas such as an anesthetic. Intranasal administration means that the drug is absorbed through your nasal passages into your bloodstream. Parenteral drug administration means that a medicine is administered in your vein, muscle or under your skin.

Drug absorption occurs when drugs are taken into your body. Drugs must readily dissolve in fat to pass through the lining of your gastrointestinal tract. The stomach is highly acidic, which favors absorption of weakly acidic drugs. The small intestine is slightly alkaline, which favors the absorption of weakly basic drugs. The small intestine is the major site of drug absorption due to its large surface area. Bioavailability describes what proportion of the administered drug is available to produce a pharmacologic response. Some factors influencing drug bioavailability include how rapidly and completely the drug will dissolve and will be absorbed through your gastrointestinal tract. Factors influencing drug bioavailability are: the presence of food may affect the dissolution and absorption of drugs, excretion in your feces, a deficiency or absence of gastric hydrochloric acid, which prevents gastric absorption of acidic drugs and prevents dissolution of basic drugs.

Drug distribution is also important for you to understand. Drug distribution means that the drug that you took ultimately has to go somewhere such as your brain heart, etc. It may go to many other areas before it gets to where you want it to go. In other words, it may go to many areas in your body. The degree of drug distribution depends on the physical and chemical properties of a drug and its ability to penetrate cell membranes, capillaries, the blood-brain barrier, placenta, etc. The Blood-Brain Barrier (BBB) surrounds your brain. Only very lipid-soluble drugs and extremely small molecules penetrate the BBB to exert an effect on your brain.

Plasma protein binding is also important because many drugs may bind reversibly with plasma proteins. Only unbound drugs may produce a pharmacologic effect and then be broken down (be metabolized) and then be excreted. Only the unbound free drug is excreted. Your drug stops working when it is metabolized. Drug metabolism occurs when liver enzymes convert lipid-soluble drugs to water-soluble breakdown products called metabolites. These metabolites are eliminated from your body by your kidneys.

Drugs pass through your stomach and small intestines and enter you liver before going into your blood stream. This is called the first-pass effect. This allows the liver to metabolize (change) some drugs before they are distributed throughout your body. Drugs can be converted into fewer active drugs by your liver. For example, hydrocodone can be converted to hydromorphone. After drug metabolism, the drug is eliminated by your kidneys. Know that the onset of action of a drug is the time, after a drug is administered; to achieve a blood concentration required to produce a detectable response like pain relief. The duration of action of a drug is the amount of time a drug is present in your body. A certain dose of drug is required to achieve a response (e.g. pain relief), and a point will be reached where increasing the drug dose will not increase the therapeutic pain relief response.

Liver enzymes that metabolize your drugs may be induced or inhibited by other drugs as well as cigarettes and cause drug-drug interactions, which mean that other drugs that you are taking may make your pain pill not work. Know that the half-life is the amount of time required for elimination processes to reduce the drug concentration in your body by one-half. The volume of distribution is the volume of your body in which a drug is distributed. The steady state occurs when the intake of a drug is in equilibrium with its elimination. In other words, what goes into your body is the amount that goes out of your body. The volume of distribution is a proportionality factor that relates the amount of drug in the body to the concentration of drug measured in a biological fluid (your serum). Think of the body as a container of water. The ingested drug is either in your blood compartment or is in your tissue. A drug is more effective if it in your blood and not in your tissues. The drug will only become efficient when it is out of your tissues and is in your blood stream. At low doses of each drug, a dosage increase results in only a small increase in drug response. At higher doses, an increase in dosage produces a much greater response.

Usually there is not a single cause why your medication may not work. The following are some reasons why your medication may not work:

1. Most drugs are manufactured for a specific ailment. If your diagnosis is wrong and if you were prescribed a specific drug for a specific disease, your drug will not work.

2. Your prescribed drug may be adversely affected by your hormones.

3. Other drugs that you are taking may interfere with your medicine. Drug-drug interactions occur when two or more drugs react with each other. Drug-food/beverage interactions result from drugs reacting with foods or beverages. Drug-condition interactions may occur when an existing medical condition makes certain drugs potentially harmful. Some drugs compete for the same receptor.

4. Your drug won't work if it is not absorbed by your stomach or small intestine due to excess acid in your stomach.

5. Many drugs will not work unless the drug is converted into a new medication in your liver. You may have a genetic mutation which prevents this conversion. A genetic test can determine this.

6. Your dose of medication may not be sufficient.

7. Your medicine may not be potent enough. You may need a stronger medication.

8. Most drugs need to be absorbed from your stomach or small intestine to enter your blood stream. Previous abdominal surgery may not leave a way for a drug to get into your blood stream.

9. Your liver may filter a large portion of the drug before it gets to the proper receptor.

10. Your kidneys may excrete your drug too quickly before it has time to give you relief.

11. Some foods that you eat may interact with your medication causing your medication not to work.

12. Smoking may inhibit the effects of some medications.

13. Many medications are divided into subclasses. A change from one subclass to another subclass may be more effective for your condition.

14. Pain and stress can also decrease the amount of drugs absorbed into your body.

15. Drug tolerance occurs when a patient develops a decreased response to a drug over time. You then require a larger dose of medication to produce the same response.

16. Some generic drugs may not work as well as the brand-name drugs.

17. Your gender may affect how your drug works.

18. Medications may be given by mouth, by patch, by suppository, by injection or by nasal spray. If one form of drug is ineffective, another form may work.

19. Some drugs compete for the same receptor (e.g. Narcan and Morphine where Narcan pushes the Morphine off the mu receptor which stops the effects of the Morphine).

20. The most common reasons why your medication will not work are related to the interactions of your drug with other drugs, foods, juices, etc.

21. You must read all the instructions and warnings that come with your medication for your drug to work effective.

## 2. Drug Metabolism

Once you take a medication, it is transformed in your body by complex chemical reactions. Drug metabolism, therefore, is the body's processing and excreting of drugs. The sum of all chemical reactions within a living body is known as metabolism. Drug metabolism is the body's way of transforming drugs, from the original chemical substance to another chemical so that they can be excreted from your body. Drug metabolism, therefore, is the process by which the body breaks down and converts medication into active chemical substances. In essence, drug metabolism, therefore, is the process by which the body changes a drug from its dosage form to a more water-soluble form that can then be excreted. Most drugs are metabolized into inactive products which are then excreted. Other drugs are converted to active metabolites, which are capable of exerting their own pharmacologic action. Hydrocodone, for example, is converted to hydromorphone, which helps to decrease your pain. Active metabolites may then undergo further metabolism or may be excreted from your body unchanged.

Drugs can interact with other drugs, foods, and beverages. The primary site of drug metabolism is the liver. Enzymes in the liver are responsible for chemically changing drug components into substances known as metabolites. Metabolite excretion is done through the kidneys. Metabolism lowers the concentration of medication in the bloodstream. The metabolic rate can vary significantly from person to person, and drug dosages that work quickly and effectively in one individual may not work well for another. Factors such as genetics, environment, nutrition, and age also influence drug metabolism; infants and elderly patients may have a reduced capacity to metabolize certain drugs, and may require adjustments in dosage.

Many drugs do not work in your body until they have been changed in your body by enzymes that transform them into chemicals that will work in your body. An analogy is chocolate milk. Chocolate syrup a chemical is added to milk to form chocolate milk. Plain milk was essentially "metabolized" to chocolate milk in a glass of milk. Most medications are altered in your body to other drugs that work in your body.

Generally, drugs are excreted by your kidneys to rid your body of these chemicals. These chemicals cannot be excreted in your urine by the kidneys until they can dissolve in water. Most of one's drug conversion to a drug or drugs that can be excreted takes place in your liver.

Genetic variation among people can greatly affect the metabolism of some drugs as well. The families of liver isoenzymes known as cytochrome P-450 enzymes are crucial to drug metabolism. These isoenzymes have a catabolic (molecular breaking down) action on medications, by breaking them down into other chemicals called metabolites. Consequently, these isoenzymes also act to lower the concentration of a medication in your bloodstream.

One of the problems with taking drugs orally is that some can be excreted from the body without even being metabolized. To avoid this, pharmaceutical companies have utilized drug design to develop chemicals what are called prodrugs. These are drugs that are initially less active or inactive, but once in the body are metabolized into an active metabolite.

Drug metabolism usually consists of two phases. Phase 1 involves introducing a chemical structure on to the drug in question that makes it water-soluble. Frequently, this reaction introduces an atom of oxygen onto the drug. This usually results in another chemical group being added to the molecule. Phase 2 metabolism consists of adding a compound that will allow the intermediate to be excreted by the kidneys. This step is called conjugation. Often, it involves adding chemicals to the drug molecule. This increases its solubility in water, so that it can be excreted from your body.

The metabolism of one drug can frequently cause an interaction with another drug. The presence of a drug can induce a greater concentration of particular enzyme that can then metabolize other drugs in the body. This leads to lowered concentrations of the other drugs. Another possibility is that the drug you are taking may directly inhibit metabolism of an alternate drug, which may lead to an excessive drug level in your body.

You need to be aware that individuals who metabolize a drug poorly may be prone to overdose even when taking a low dose of the drug. On the other hand, extensive metabolizers of a drug may need a higher dosage of the drug to obtain a therapeutic effect and consequently, your drug may not work for you. Your physician can do genetic testing in many instances to determine what type of drug metabolizer that you are. You will then be prescribed the appropriate medication.

## 3. Drug Interactions

A drug interaction is a situation in which another drug or any substances, including food that can affect the activity of a drug that you are currently taking. A drug interaction occurs when a substance affects the activity of a drug. The effects of the drug that you are taking may be increased or decreased or not affected at all. Drug interactions may make your drug less effective, cause unexpected side effects, or increase the action of a particular drug. Some drug interactions can even be harmful to you. Interactions between drugs are called drug-drug interactions. However, interactions may also exist between drugs and foods such as grapefruit juice, and some medications that you are taking. These occurrences may occur out of accidental misuse or due to lack of knowledge about the ingredients involved in some substances. Interactions can lessen or magnify the desired therapeutic effect of a drug, or may cause unwanted or unexpected side effects.

A drug interaction, therefore, is an occurrence where a substance affects the activity of a drug when both are administered together. This action is synergistic when a drug's effect is increased or antagonistic where a drug's effect is decreased. Occasionally, a new effect can be produced by a drug that neither drug produces on its own.

Drug interactions may also occur between drugs and foods as well as drugs and herbs. Patients taking some antidepressant drugs should not take food containing tyramine as an individual's blood pressure may become extremely elevated. A hypertensive crisis may occur. These interactions may occur to lack of knowledge about the ingredients involved in drugs or foods. Over-the-counter drug labels also contain information about ingredients, uses, warnings and directions that is important to read and understand. Drug tolerance occurs when a patient develops a decreased response to a drug over time. You will then require larger doses to produce the same response.

Your pharmacist will warn you about potential serious drug interaction that is possible when you take a certain drug. For example, chocolate; alcoholic beverages, cheese, sour cream, yogurt, soy sauce, sauerkraut, beans, snow peas, bananas, pineapple, eggplants, figs, red plums, raspberries, nuts, and processed meats must be avoided when taking some antidepressants. Your prescribing physician and pharmacist will warn you about which foods to avoid with certain depression medications.

The factors or conditions that predispose you one to drug interactions include: elderly patients, taking many medications, genetics, and kidney and liver diseases. Older individuals may have factors relating to how human physiology changes with age may affect the effect of some drugs. For example, liver metabolism, kidney function and nerve transmission decrease with age. Each of these factors can increase the chances of errors being made in the administration of drugs.

The more drugs that you take, will make it more likely it will be that some or all of them will interact and ultimately cause you to have potential severe drug or even fatal drug reactions. Genes, predominantly in your liver synthesize enzymes. These enzymes break down drugs that you take. Some enzymes however, have genetic variations that could decrease or increase the activity of these enzymes. The consequence of this would, on occasions, be a greater predisposition towards drug interactions and therefore a greater predisposition for adverse effects to occur.

This occurrence is seen in variations in your liver cytochrome P450 enzymes (CYPs). CYPs are the enzymes involved in drug metabolism. Most drugs undergo deactivation by CYPs. Also, many substances are transformed by CYPs to form their active compounds. An example is hydrocodone, which is a pain medication. Hydrocodone is transformed to hydromorphone, which is a pain medication. Your CYPs are involved in this transformation. Without this conversion to hydromorphone, you would have minimal or no pain relief.

Liver and kidney diseases can affect your drug blood levels. The blood concentrations of drugs that are metabolized in the liver and or eliminated by the kidneys may be altered if either of these organs is not functioning correctly. If this is the case, an increase in blood concentrations may be markedly elevated, which could cause you to have a drug overdose.

When an interaction between two drugs causes an increase in the effects of one or both of the drugs this interaction is called a synergistic effect. Alcohol, for example, will potentiate the effect of pain pills. Two drugs are additive if half of each drug given together produces the same effect as the full dose of either drug alone. This is also called an additive effect. Codeine and acetaminophen (Tylenol) for example, may have additive effects. If the response of the two drugs at half of the usual dose is greater than the full dose of either drug, the two drugs are said to be synergistic.

Some drug interactions can even be harmful to you. Reading the label every time you use a nonprescription or prescription drug and taking the time to learn about drug interactions may be critical to your health. Drug interactions may occur when an existing medical condition makes certain drugs potentially harmful. For example, if you have high blood pressure, you could experience an unwanted hypertensive reaction if you take a nasal decongestant.

Always tell your pharmacist what prescribed or nonprescribed medication that you are taking. Before taking a drug, ask your doctor or pharmacist the following questions: Can I take it with other drugs? Should I avoid certain foods, beverages or other products? What are possible drug interaction signs I should know about? How will the drug work in my body?

Always read your drug labels, including any over the counter drugs that you may be taking. Over-the-counter drug labels should contain information about ingredients, uses, warnings and directions that is important for you to read and understand. The label also includes important information about possible drug interactions. As previously stated, you have to remember to read the labels on your drug bottles and or packages before taking any drug!

## 4. Gender Factor

Men and women may respond differently to medications and therefore respond to treatments differently. For example, most women have a lower tolerance for pain than men do and are more sensitive and likely to express their feelings of pain than men. Female sex has been shown to be a risk factor for clinically relevant adverse drug reactions. Generally, males weigh more than females, yet few drugs are dosed based on body weight. Pharmacologic changes between sexes can affect both the desired therapeutic effect of a drug as well as its adverse effects profiles.

For example, most clinical pain disorders are more common in women than in men, particularly during the peak reproductive years. This suggests that fluctuations in the ovarian hormones encountered during the female menstrual cycle may increase pain responses. There are gender differences in the pharmacokinetics and/or pharmacodynamics of drugs as well. One obvious reason for these differences is that women tend to have a lower body weight than men. Adults are often given the same dose of drug as previously regardless of body weight, so women tend to have higher serum concentrations of drugs than men.

The causes and treatment of pain may be different for men and women. Considerable evidence indicates sex-related differences in pain responses and in the effectiveness of various pain medications. One of the reasons men and women feel pain differently has to do with the effect of sex hormones on pain receptors in the brain and spinal cord. There is a substantial body of evidence suggesting that the sex hormones, particularly estradiol and progesterone, play a role in pain perception. Women respond more favorably to a class of antidepressant medications called serotonin-specific reuptake inhibitors, or SSRIs, than to other antidepressants known as tricyclics. Although hormones are not the only reason a drug or medication might affect men and women differently, the question of hormonal influences on drug responses may be critical for the addiction field

Gender differences are important with respect to drug action, especially because the menstrual cycle can affect the amount of medication in the blood (blood levels) related to excess body fluid noted during the menstrual cycle. If a female retains fluid, the excess fluid will dilute the action of a drug. Nalbuphine, pentazocine, and butorphanol, mixed agonist/antagonist opioids that induce analgesia by acting predominantly at kappa opioid receptors, have been shown in single dose studies to have greater analgesic efficacy in women than in men.

Morphine, a mu receptor agonist has greater efficacy in male in animal studies.

Women are more than twice as likely to be diagnosed with depression and may also report more atypical and anxiety symptoms than men. Gender effects differ in the metabolism and distribution of antidepressants. Women have more side effects with antidepressant-type medications than men. They suffer more fatigue, gastrointestinal effects, and other adverse effects than men. Gonadal hormonal changes in women that occur monthly (before, during and after the menstrual cycle) alter the metabolism of certain drugs and can affect their removal from the body. One of the reasons why affects differ in the perception of pain results from the effects of the female hormones estrogen and progesterone on the brain and spinal cord.

The effects of the menstrual cycle on the nervous system vary before, during, and after menses. Male and female brains have approximately the same number of receptors for estrogen and androgen. Researchers concluded that gender-specific hormone, and hormonal receptor differences also influence the regulation and transmission of the nervous impulses that transmit pain.

Estrogen a female hormone, affects the central nervous system levels of dopamine and serotonin, which when decreased affect mood disorders and usually cause depression. Men and women also differ in the metabolism and distribution of antidepressants and the presence of estrogen in women of childbearing age may interfere with the mechanism of action of a number of antidepressants. These differences have led many researchers to question whether antidepressants are equally effective and tolerated in men and women. Women experience more depression than males. Men may have more serotonin receptors, which may be a reason why they suffer from a lower incidence of depression. As a result, a woman's greater sensitivity to pain may be dependent on the fact that she has fewer serotonins in the brain and spinal cord.

Some pain syndromes are affected by changes in sex hormones. For example, migraine headaches resolve during pregnancy as a result of elevated blood levels of progesterone. When estrogen decreases, in some patients, joint pains increase in females. In men, a decrease in testosterone will increase the frequency of angina. With an increase in testosterone, cluster headaches are more prevalent in men. With an increase in progesterone, testosterone, and estrogen, both men and women experience an increase in temporomandibular joint pain.

Drug metabolism may differ in men and women. Liver enzymes in women may also not metabolize the antidepressants of the selective serotonin-specific reuptake inhibitor class. Pentazocine (a kappa stimulating analgesic) produces significantly greater analgesia in females than in males. The reason for this observation remains to be elucidated.

There are notable sex differences in the incidence and manifestations of virtually all central nervous system disorders, including neurodegenerative disease (Parkinson's and Alzheimer's), chronic pain, drug abuse, anxiety, and depression. Male and female nervous systems respond differently to traumatic brain injury and in vivo research relates this difference to neuroprotection from female sex hormones.

Gender may be an important variable in the processes of absorption, distribution, metabolism, and excretion of drugs taken by males and females. Women have a lower stomach acid secretion than men. This can increase the absorption of drugs such as Elavil or Valium, and decrease the absorption of acidic drugs such as dilantin and barbiturates. Women weigh less than men and have a lower total blood value than men. Body fat is 11 percent higher in women between the ages of 25 and 35, which can increase the volume of distribution of many drugs. This means that the drug prescribed is stored in tissue.

Opioid therapy efficacy can decrease in both men and women if serum testosterone (a male hormone) levels decrease. Testosterone therapy may normalize hormone levels and improve a number of quality of life parameters (e.g., sexual function, well-being, and mood) in men and women.

Gender differences in antidepressant treatments, including responses and side effects, have been studied. Women may better respond to selective serotonin reuptake inhibitors (Celexa) than tricyclic antidepressants (amitriptyline). Men responded better to a tricyclic antidepressant (amitriptyline) than to a selective serotonin reuptake inhibitor. Women taking selective serotonin reuptake inhibitors are more likely to report side effects of nausea and dizziness, whereas men reported increased urinary frequency and sexual dysfunction.

Compression of the median nerve in the carpal tunnel is a common compression neuropathy. This entity affects women more than men. The average age at the onset of this ailment is between 40 and 60 years of age. Carpal tunnel syndrome (CTS) patients are known to show gender-related differences in severity as well.

Osteoarthritis is 2-3 times more prevalent in females than males. Osteoarthritis, which affects 40 percent of middle-age patients and approximately 70 percent of geriatric patients, essentially will have the same degree of input into the central nervous system of men and women. Osteoporosis can be a significant bone disease because it is potentially disabling. Approximately 30 percent of all postmenopausal Caucasian women will suffer from fractures related to osteoporosis. Even though osteoporosis is a disease that mostly affects women, osteoporosis can be seen in a small percentage of men as well.

Fibromyalgia (FM) is a chronic pain syndrome that affects soft tissue, tendons, and fascia. It affects about 5 percent of the population, 90 percent of which are women of childbearing age. Male patients with FM had fever symptoms and fewer TP, and less common "hurt all over," fatigue, morning fatigue, and IBS, compared with female patients. Myofascial trigger points occur when there is trauma to a muscle or prolonged tension in a muscle from faulty posture. With respect to gender specificity, it appears that men suffer more from acute myofascial pain, whereas women suffer more from latent myofascial pain syndromes. Latent myofascial trigger points are more prevalent in women who are not active with respect to aerobic exercise. On the other hand, active trigger points are more prevalent in men who are doing vigorous exercises or who are doing heavy manual labor.

Temporomandibular joint (TMJ) dysfunction prevalence peaks between the ages of 25 and 44. TMJ dysfunction pain is less in males versus females but also shows that testosterone reduces TMJ pain at supra physiological serum levels.

Female gender is associated with about a 40% lower rate of myocardial infarction. Anginal chest pain in men may spread to the jaws and arms. Numbness and pain radiating from the chest into the left arm is especially characteristic of anginal pain in men. In women with a decrease in oxygen to the heart muscle for some reason, symptoms of angina pain include pressure in the center of the chest accompanied by pain in the neck or arms.

The distribution of Complex Regional Pain Syndrome (CRPS) between men and women is almost equal for individuals younger than 50 years of age. However, for those over 50 years of age there is a predominance of CRPS noted in women. Complex Regional Pain Syndrome (CRPS) usually develops after a noxious event, but spontaneous onsets, mostly in females have been described in 3-11% of the cases. Additional research is needed to clarify the mechanisms for sex differences in pain as well as responses to pain treatments and to develop new treatment modalities that improve pain management for both men and women. The "one size fits all" mentality is no longer acceptable.

## 5. Generic or Brand Name?

In general, new brand-name drugs are costly. Prescription costs are a common health care cost for many people and also the source of considerable economic hardship for some people. Generic drugs are less expensive. This is because drug development affects the price of a drug and is the process of bringing a drug to the pharmaceutical market. A generic drug is a drug that is comparable to a brand drug product in dosage form, strength, quality and performance characteristics, and intended use. Generic drugs are nearly identical or within an acceptable bioequivalent range to its brand-name counterpart. Generic drugs are equivalent to the brand formulation if they have the same active substance, the same pharmaceutical form and the same therapeutic indications and a similar bioequivalence respect to the reference medicinal product.

The time it takes a generic drug to appear on the market varies. It is usually 20 years. Generic drugs are usually sold for significantly lower prices than their branded equivalents. A generic drug refers to any drug marketed under its chemical name without advertising but the company that made the drug. New drugs may be initially tested on animals. The new drug is then evaluated in human clinical trials. Eventually, the drug's patent will expire, and the drug becomes a generic drug. Clinical trials for new drugs involve four steps: Phase I trials, usually in healthy volunteers, to determine safety and dosing. Phase II trials are used to explore safety in small numbers of sick patients. Phase III trials are large trials to determine safety and efficacy in sufficiently sizeable numbers of patients. Finally Phase IV trials are post FDA approval trials that are called post-market surveillance studies, which attempt that the drugs work and cause no serious side effect to patients over time.

The full cost of bringing a new drug can amount to hundreds of millions or even billions of dollars. It has been reported that it takes approximately $800 million to bring one new drug from the original study phase to market. Careful decision making during a new drug development by a pharmaceutical company is therefore, essential to avoid costly failures to the drug company. Well-designed studies and comparisons against both a placebo (a pill with no medication) with a gold-standard treatment play a major role in achieving reliable drug effect data.

Historically, drugs were discovered through identifying the active ingredient from traditional remedies. For example, aspirin was discovered from Willow bark to relieve joint pain in the late 1800's in Germany. Your drug will not work unless it goes to a target. The target is the cellular or molecular structure that the drug-in-development is meant to act on. The majority of targets currently selected for drug discovery efforts are proteins.

The ideal scenario is to find a molecule which will interfere with only the chosen target, but not other, related targets.

The first step in the development of drugs is the discovery of a new compound that affects a medical condition. The new drug must be safe and effective in animals. Step 2 involves testing in a small number of healthy human volunteers to confirm the information from the animal studies is the same in humans and to gain further information on the effects of the new drug. Finally, the new compound is tested in humans who have the condition for which it will be used. Once the compound is proven to be safe and effective for the condition, or disease the company applies to the Food and Drug Administration (FDA) for a license to manufacture and sell this drug.

Drug companies are like other companies in that they manufacture products that must be sold for a profit in order for the company to survive and grow. Much expense is incurred in the early phases of development of compounds by drug companies that will not become approved drugs. In addition, it takes about 7 to 10 years and an average cost of 500 million dollars to develop each new drug. If the drug is not approved by the FDA, the company loses the money. These expenses must be covered by the revenue from new drugs that successfully become approved drugs.

After a drug is approved, millions of dollars are spent on marketing in educating healthcare providers and conducting post-marketing studies. Drug companies spend a lot of money on marketing because of competition they face from other drug companies for their drugs. In addition to maximizing returns on their investment through advertising, drug companies also spend money to find new uses for drugs or better ways of using them. These efforts increase the use of the approved drugs and also benefit patients.

The price paid by a patient for a medication must cover the costs of developing new compounds that become approved drugs and compounds that fail to become drugs, as well as marketing, post-marketing studies, and a profit. Without the promise of a reasonable profit, there is very little incentive for any company to develop new drugs. There is no denying that drugs are expensive. However, the price of drugs should be weighed against their benefits. Many drugs reduce pain and sufferings, prevent disease, or extend life.

Medications are assigned to one of four categories known as coinsurance tiers, based on drug usage, cost and clinical effectiveness. A higher Tier is more expensive than a lower Tier. Copayment Definitions for the Four-Tier Enhanced Formulary are as follows: Tier 1. Generic Drugs: Features the lowest copayment. Tier 2. Preferred Brand-Name Drugs:

Preferred brand-name products are based on safety, efficacy and cost and have the second lowest copayment. Tier 3. These drugs are Non-Preferred Brand-Name Drugs and Preferred Specialty Drugs. This Tier usually includes non-preferred brand name medications. Tier 4. Specialty Drugs are medications which require special dosing or administration are typically prescribed by a specialist and are more expensive than most medications and have the highest copayment or coinsurance amounts.Brand-name drugs for which alternatives are available in Tier 1 or Tier 2 and are not used as a first line of patient treatment. Preferred specialty brand-name drugs have higher copayments.

    Pharmacologically, generic medications have been tested and should provide the same results as brand name drugs. You may not have been prescribed the appropriate drug whether or not it is generic or brand name. You may also be experiencing a drug-drug interaction where one drug negates the effects of another drug. Patients should remember that all drugs go through the Food and Drug Administration whether it is a generic medicine or a branded medication. Medications in the market go through a series of examinations to ensure that they're safe for human consumption. Therefore, generic medications s should work as well as branded ones.

## 6. What is a Scheduled Drug?

The Comprehensive Drug Abuse Prevention and Control Act were made law in 1970. Title II of this law, the Controlled Substances Act, is the legal foundation of narcotics enforcement in the United States. The Comprehensive Drug Abuse Prevention and Control Act were made law in 1970. Title II of this law, the Controlled Substances Act, is the legal foundation of narcotics enforcement in the United States. The Comprehensive Drug Abuse Prevention and Control Act were made law in 1970. Title II of this law, the Controlled Substances Act, is the legal foundation of narcotics enforcement in the United States.

The Controlled Substances Act (CSA) is the statute prescribing federal U.S. drug policy under which the manufacture, importation, possession, use and distribution of certain substances are regulated. It was passed by the 91st United States Congress as Title II of the Comprehensive Drug Abuse Prevention and Control Act of 1970 and signed into law by President Richard Nixon. The legislation created five Schedules (classifications), with varying qualifications for a substance to be included in each.

The Controlled Substances Act consists of 2 subchapters. Subchapter I defines Schedules I-V, lists chemicals used in the manufacture of controlled substances, and differentiates lawful and unlawful manufacturing, distribution, and possession of controlled substances, including possession of Schedule I drugs for personal use.

Drugs, substances, and certain chemicals used to make drugs are classified into five distinct categories or schedules depending upon the drug's acceptable medical use and the drug's abuse or dependency potential. The abuse rate is a determinate factor in the scheduling of the drug; for example, Schedule I drugs are considered the most dangerous class of drugs with a high potential for abuse and potentially severe psychological and/or physical dependence.

As the drug schedule changes, Schedule II, Schedule III, etc., so does the abuse potential. Schedule V drugs represent the least potential for abuse. A Listing of drugs and their schedule are located at Controlled Substance Act (CSA) Scheduling or CSA Scheduling by Alphabetical Order. These lists describe the basic or parent chemical and do not necessarily describe the salts, isomers and salts of isomers, esters, ethers and derivatives, which may also be classified as controlled substances. These lists are intended as general references and are not comprehensive listings of all controlled substances.

Please note that a substance needs not be listed as a controlled substance to be treated as a Schedule I substance for criminal prosecution. A controlled substance analogue is a substance which is intended for human consumption and is structurally or pharmacologically substantially similar to or is represented as being similar to a Schedule I or Schedule II substance and is not an approved medication in the United States.

Schedule I

Schedule I drugs, substances, or chemicals are defined as drugs with no currently accepted medical use and a high potential for abuse. Schedule I drugs are the most dangerous drugs of all the drug schedules with potentially severe psychological or physical dependence. Some examples of Schedule I drugs are: heroin, lysergic acid diethylamide (LSD), marijuana (cannabis), 3, 4-methylenedioxymethamphetamine (ecstasy), methaqualone, and peyote. No prescriptions may be written for Schedule I substances.

Schedule II

Schedule II drugs, substances, or chemicals are defined as drugs with a high potential for abuse, less abuse potential than Schedule I drugs, with use potentially leading to severe psychological or physical dependence. These drugs are also considered dangerous. Some examples of Schedule II drugs are: Combination products with less than 15 milligrams of hydrocodone per dosage unit (Vicodin), cocaine, methamphetamine, methadone, hydromorphone (Dilaudid), meperidine (Demerol), oxycodone (OxyContin), fentanyl, Dexedrine, Adderall, and Ritalin.

Schedule III

Schedule III drugs, substances, or chemicals are defined as drugs with a moderate to low potential for physical and psychological dependence. Schedule III drugs abuse potential is less than Schedule I and Schedule II drugs but more than Schedule IV. Some examples of Schedule III drugs are: products containing less than 90 milligrams of codeine per dosage unit (Tylenol with codeine), ketamine, anabolic steroids, and testosterone.

Schedule IV

Schedule IV drugs, substances, or chemicals are defined as drugs with a low potential for abuse and low risk of dependence. Some examples of Schedule IV drugs are: Xanax, Soma, Valium, Ativan, Talwin, Ambien, Tramadol.

Schedule V

Schedule V drugs, substances, or chemicals are defined as drugs with lower potential for abuse than Schedule IV and consist of preparations containing limited quantities of certain narcotics. Schedule V drugs are generally used for antidiarrheal, antitussive, and analgesic purposes. Some examples of Schedule V drugs are: cough preparations with less than 200 milligrams of codeine or per 100 milliliters (Robitussin AC), Lomotil, Motofen, Lyrica, Parepectolin.

## 7. How Drugs are made

A pharmaceutical drug also referred to as a medicinal drug is a substance used to treat disease. Drugs are substances derived mostly from plants. Some of the plants are edible plants while some are poisonous plants. Pharmaceutical companies take only the active ingredient from the plant, making the natural ingredient unnatural. However, a natural ingredient that is altered chemically can be patented. This depends on the drug in question. Most drugs are derived from plants. Marijuana is prepared from the Cannabis plant. Cocaine is synthesized from the coca plant. On the other hand, some drugs are produced artificially. Methamphetamine, for example, is an artificial drug that is engineered chemically.

Early medicine was a process of soaking herbs in water or alcohol to extract the active ingredients which were then drunk as a tea. As methods progressed, it was found that the dried herbs could be used and that, by powdering the dried herb, a small amount of the powder could be taken thus forgoing the need to make a tea. Various herbs could be mixed together and swallowed with water. They could also be mixed with minerals and chemicals that were found to have medicinal properties. Methods were eventually found to extract the medicinally active parts of plants and manufactured them as powders.

When a virus enters our body, it tries to attack a cell. Once inside the cell, the virus can hijack the cell's own replication machinery, which starts to make many copies of the virus. These viruses burst out of the cell, destroying it, and will attempt to infect many more cells unless tackled by the immune system. The infection can also start to spread to other people. An influenza vaccine is made up of parts of an inactive influenza virus or a version of the virus which doesn't have the ability to cause an infection. Antiviral drugs are mostly chemical in nature and can be synthesized in a large scale. They are designed to inhibit viruses from replicating in your body. The immune response leads to something called acquired immunity. Your body remembers viruses so that it can quickly destroy them, should they return.

A pharmaceutical drug is a drug used to diagnose, cure, treat, or prevent disease. Drugs are classified on the basis of their origin: 1. Drug from natural origin: Herbal or plant or mineral origin, some drug substances are of marine origin. 2. Drug from chemical as well as natural origin. 3. Some drugs are derived from chemical synthesis. 4. Other drugs are derived from animal origin such as hormones, and enzymes. 5. Drug can also be derived from microbial origin to make antibiotics.

Microorganisms are living organisms that are too small to be seen individually by the naked eye viewed. They include bacteria, viruses, protozoa, and some fungi and algae. Antimicrobials are products that kill microorganisms or keep them from multiplying (reproducing) or growing. They are most commonly used to prevent or treat disease and infections due to microorganisms. Antibiotics are substances that are actually produced by one microorganism and have the ability to kill or inhibit the growth or reproduction of other microorganisms. The vast majority of antibiotics are used primarily to kill or inhibit the growth of bacteria. Antibiotics are subdivided into two categories, broad spectrum and narrow spectrum, based on the number and types of bacteria they affect. Broad-spectrum antibiotics are effective against many types of bacteria, while narrow spectrum antibiotics are effective against a more limited range of bacteria. Anti-viral drugs and anti-fungal drugs are also antimicrobials, but they are not antibiotics. Antimicrobial resistance and antibiotic resistance occur when a microorganism develops the ability to resist the action of an antimicrobial.

In general, many tablets or capsules usually contain additives that aid in the manufacturing process or in how the medication pill is accepted by your body. Cellulose, lactose, calcium, or dextrin is added to many medications as a filler, to give the medicine proper bulk. Modified cellulose gum or starch is often added to vitamins as a disintegration agent. That is, it helps the vitamin compound break up once it is ingested. Vitamin tablets are also usually coated, to give the tablets a particular color or flavor, or to determine how the tablet is absorbed (in the stomach versus in the intestine, slowly versus all at once, etc.). Many coatings are made from a cellulose base. An additional coating of carnauba wax is often put on as well, to give the tablet a polished appearance.

A pharmaceutical company purchases raw ingredients from distributors. In many cases, the manufacturer will, nevertheless, test the raw materials or send samples to an independent laboratory for analysis. These substances may be tested for possible bacterial contamination as well. Laboratory technicians verify that all the ingredients of a medication are distributed in the same proportion throughout the mix. The finished medication mixture can be compressed into tablets, sometimes with a coating, or encapsulated in preformed gelatin capsules. These substances are inspected again before they are packaged and then are sent to pharmacies, clinics hospitals, etc.

Like pills, topical medications have to have a stringent manufacturing standard as well. A topical medication is a medication that is applied to body surfaces such as the skin or mucous membranes to treat ailments via a large range of classes, including but not limited to creams, foams, gels, lotions, and ointments.

Some animal parts are used to make drugs. The gelatin coatings, capsules and liquid additives for medicines are not made from harmless food, but rather from the skin, cartilage, connective tissues and bones of animals.

Drug products topically administered via the skin fall into two general categories; those applied for local action and those for systemic effects. Common products in the former category include creams, gels, ointments, pastes, suspensions, lotions, foams, sprays, aerosols, and solutions. The most common drug products applied to the skin for systemic effects are referred to as self-adhering transdermal drug-delivery systems (TDS) or transdermal patches. A common example is the fentanyl pain patch.

Two categories of tests, product quality tests and product performance tests are performed on topical drug products to provide assurances of batch-to-batch quality, reproducibility, reliability, and performance.

Creams are semisolid dosage forms that contain one or more drug substances dissolved or dispersed in a suitable base. Emulsions are viscid, multiphase systems in which one or more liquids are dispersed throughout another immiscible liquid in the form of small droplets. Foams are emulsified systems packaged in pressurized containers or special dispensing devices that contain dispersed gas bubbles, usually in a liquid continuous phase, that when dispensed has a fluffy, semisolid consistency. Gels are semisolid systems consisting of either suspensions composed of small inorganic particles or large organic molecules interpenetrated by a liquid. Although the term lotion may be applied to a solution, lotions usually are fluid, somewhat viscid emulsion dosage forms for external application to the skin. Ointments are semisolids intended for external application. They serve to keep medicaments in prolonged contact with the skin and act as occlusive dressings to the skin or mucous membranes. Pastes are semisolid dosage forms that contain a high percentage (often 50%) of finely dispersed solids with a stiff consistency intended for topical application. Powders are solids or mixture of solids in a dry, finely divided state for external use. Sprays are products formed by the generation of droplets of solution containing dissolved drug for application to the skin or mucous membranes. Transdermal delivery systems (TDS) are self-contained, discrete dosage forms that, when applied to intact skin, are designed to deliver the drug(s) through the skin to the systemic circulation.

Product quality tests must be done for topical drugs not unlike oral drugs. Tube uniformity tests for topical drugs in tubes should be done to ensure that the amount of drug is the same at the top, middle and bottom of a tube of medication. A test that is discriminating and capable of detecting a sudden drug release, such as leakage, from the transdermal system should be performed before the drug is marketed. Fentanyl is more potent than morphine and a sudden leak of the drug from its system could be lethal. Lotions are similar to solutions but are thicker and tend to be more emollient in nature than solution. A tincture is a skin preparation that has a high percentage of alcohol.

If you have allergies to chemicals, food colors, animal parts, etc. read the label on your medication bottle.

## 8. Herbal "Drugs"

An herb is a plant or plant part used for its scent, flavor, or therapeutic properties. Herbal medicines are one type of dietary supplement. They are sold as tablets, capsules, powders, teas, extracts, and fresh or dried plants. People use herbal medicines to try to maintain or improve their health.

Plants have been used for medicinal purposes long before recorded history. Ancient Chinese and Egyptian papyrus writings describe medicinal uses for plants as early as 3,000 BC. The World Health Organization estimated that 80% of people worldwide rely on herbal medicines for some part of their primary health care.

The FDA has issued a public health advisory concerning many of the herbal drug interactions. For example, some of these interactions include: Kava has been linked to liver toxicity. Kava has been taken off the market in several countries because of liver toxicity. Valerian may cause sleepiness, and in some people, it may even have the unexpected effect of overstimulating instead of sedating. Garlic, ginkgo, feverfew, and ginger, among other herbs, may increase the risk of bleeding. Evening primrose may increase the risk of seizures in people who have seizure disorders and bleeding in people with bleeding disorders or who take blood-thinning medications, such as warfarin (Coumadin).

Many people believe that products labeled "natural" are always safe and good for them. This is not true. Herbal medicines do not have to go through the testing that drugs do. Some herbs, such as comfrey and ephedra, can cause serious harm. Some herbs can interact with prescription or over-the-counter medicines. These substances may be natural, but they aren't necessarily natural to the human body.

Hundreds of herbal products and supplements are available. They are advertised to treat just about any symptom. However, there isn't a lot of trustworthy evidence to support the vast majority of these advertising claims. Some of the most popular herbal products and supplements include chondroitin sulfate, echinacea, garlic, ginkgo biloba, ginseng, glucosamine, kava, melatonin, phytoestrogens, saw palmetto, and St. John's wort.

Herbal products and supplements may not be safe if you have certain health problems. if you have any of the following health problems: blood clotting problems: cancer, diabetes, enlarged prostate gland, seizures, glaucoma, coronary artery disease, hypertension, Parkinson's disease, liver disease, stroke or thyroid disease you may want to avoid herbal substances.

Marijuana is a green, brown or gray mixture of dried, shredded leaves, stems, seeds and flowers of the hemp plant Cannabis sativa. The main active chemical in marijuana is THC (delta-9-tetrahydrocannabinol). Certain areas in the brain have a higher concentration of cannabinoid receptors. Marijuana may be effective in decreasing cancer pain in some individuals.

In the United States, the Controlled Substances Act (CSA) of 1990 classifies marijuana as a Schedule I substance, which has no approved medical use and has a high potential for abuse. However, some US states have legalized the use of marijuana or medical or recreational use. Prescription medicines containing synthetic cannabinoids (THC) are already available. Marinol (dronabinol) and Cesamet (nabilone) are synthetic cannabinoids. Both medications are used to treat chemotherapy patients who have nausea, vomiting and loss of appetite.

Marijuana has also been used for glaucoma to lower intraocular pressure (IOP), but research does not show that marijuana has a better effect than currently approved glaucoma medications. Marijuana is not FDA-approved for use in glaucoma, and may lead to other side effects such as increased heart rate and lowered blood pressure. Marijuana may increase the risk of bleeding when taken with drugs that increase the risk of bleeding. Some examples include aspirin, anticoagulants (blood thinners) such as warfarin or heparin, antiplatelet drugs such as clopidogrel and nonsteroidal anti-inflammatory drugs such as ibuprofen or naproxen. Marijuana may affect blood sugar levels. Caution is advised when using diabetic medications that may also affect blood sugar. Adverse effects of THC can occur during pregnancy and breastfeeding as well.

THC can cross the placenta. THC can depress the fetal heart rates. Studies have found that babies born to mothers who used marijuana during pregnancy were smaller than those born to mothers who did not use the drug. A nursing mother who uses marijuana passes some of the THC to the baby in her breast milk. Research indicates that use by a mother during the first month of breast-feeding can impair the infant's motor development.

Marijuana contains some of the same, and sometimes even more, of the cancer-causing chemicals found in cigarette smoke. Shortly after smoking marijuana the heart rate increases drastically and may remain elevated for up to 3 hours. The risk of heart attack may increase by up to 4.8-fold in the first hour after smoking marijuana. The effect may be due to the increased heart rate, as well as altered heart rhythms.

As of July 2014, 23 states and the District of Columbia legally allow marijuana for personal medical use. Rules surrounding the use of medical marijuana vary by state. The first state in the union to legalize the medical use of marijuana was California in 1996. Other states that allow medical marijuana include: Alaska, Arizona, California, Colorado, Connecticut, Delaware, Hawaii, Illinois, Maine, Maryland, Massachusetts, Michigan, Minnesota, Montana, Nevada, New Hampshire, New Jersey, New Mexico, New York, Oregon, Rhode Island, Vermont, Washington, and the District of Columbia. It is important to recognize that these state marijuana laws do not change the fact that using marijuana continues to be an offense under Federal law.

Some herbal remedies have the potential to cause adverse drug interactions when used in combination with various prescription and over-the-counter pharmaceuticals, and a patient should inform a herbalist of their consumption of orthodox prescription and other medications.

There are eight medical conditions for which patients can use cannabis in most states: cancer, glaucoma, HIV/AIDS, muscle spasms, seizures, severe pain, severe nausea, dramatic weight loss and muscle wasting.

Some herbal supplements, especially those imported from Asian countries, may contain high levels of heavy metals, including lead, mercury, and cadmium. It is important to purchase herbal supplements from reputable manufacturers to ensure quality. Many herbs can interact with prescription medications and cause unwanted or dangerous reactions as well.

Many of the pharmaceuticals currently available to physicians have a long history of use as herbal remedies, including opium, aspirin, digitalis, and quinine. However, adulteration, inappropriate formulation, or lack of understanding of plant and drug interactions have led to adverse reactions that are sometimes life threatening or lethal.

## 9. Drug Laws in the United States

Your medicine may not work if you take a counterfeit (a copy of a drug, in order to defraud or deceive people) drug. The Federal Government attempts to prevent counterfeit as well as designer drugs from getting into circulation. Laws are important as controlled drugs need to be regulated closely. In the United States, the first drug law was passed in San Francisco in 1875, banning the smoking of opium in opium dens. This law was aimed at controlling use among Chinese immigrants. In the 1830,'s a law was introduced in Massachusetts, which was the first law to limit alcohol availability in the U.S. This law forbade selling alcohol to Indians. Between 1851 and 1855, 13 states passed alcohol prohibition laws. By 1868, nine states repealed them. These laws, however, were addressed at those who were involved in alcohol use rather than on the alcohol itself.

In the USA, the Harrison Act was passed in 1914, and required sellers of opiates and cocaine to get a license. This Act was originally intended to regulate the drug trade, but it became a law that prohibited the sale of these substances. It soon became law that any prescription for a narcotic written by a physician or given by a pharmacist constituted a conspiracy to violate the Harrison Act. In 1919, the Supreme Court ruled that the Harrison Act was constitutional and that physicians could not prescribe narcotics solely for drug maintenance. If a physician provided a prescription of a narcotic for an addict, that physician was subject to criminal prosecution. Substances such as heroin, morphine, and cocaine were readily available in the United States and sold as part of "patent" medicines to cure everything from menstrual cramps to toothaches in children.

In 1906, the Food and Drug Act was established that affected misbranded foods and drugs. The primary concern of this law was patent medicines. Some of these compounds were made of tar, animal secretions, cocaine, heroin, etc. As far as this Act was concerned, the patent medicine could contain all or any of these substances as long as it was labeled properly.

In 1912, The Hague Conventions requested the international regulation of opium. At this time, the United States did not have any drug restrictions. Subsequently, the Harrison Tax Act was enacted in 1914. The Harrison Tax Act was a tax and only a tax. Under the act drugs obtained by addicts were to be obtained from government registered physicians.

By 1936, all 48 states regulated the sale or possession of marijuana. In 1937, the Marijuana Tax Act was instituted. State laws then made marijuana illegal.

In 1938, the Food, Drug and Cosmetic Act were instituted. The 1938 Act was enacted saying that drugs or cosmetics had to be tested for toxicity before marketing. Furthermore, adequate directions for drug or cosmetic uses needed to be on a package.

The Kefauver-Harris Amendments of 1962 stated that a drug had to be effective for what it was intended, and that approval had to be given from the government before trials on humans could be conducted. The approval came from the newly formed Food and Drug Administration. The federal government was now responsible for the safety and effectiveness of a product.

In 1965, the Drug-Abuse Control Amendments declared amphetamines, barbiturates and LSD to be dangerous drugs and allowed for FDA to recommend that these drugs be tightly controlled.

In 1972, the Federal Government recommended that marijuana to be downgraded to a misdemeanor for possession. The Carter administration worked toward Federal decriminalization of marijuana possession.

The Drug Analogue Act was enacted in 1984 to investigate designer drugs and to prevent these substances from getting to the general public. Criminals were avoiding prosecution with chemically altered versions of controlled substances with similar drug effects because they didn't appear on any of the five drug Schedules. The Anti-drug abuse act of 1986 focused on penalties for trafficking designer drugs.

The Comprehensive Methamphetamine Control Act of 1996 restricts access to chemicals and equipment used in the manufacture of methamphetamine. The Combat Meth Act of 2005 amended the Controlled Substances Act to make pseudoephedrine (the active ingredient in Sudafed and a necessary ingredient for home meth production) a Schedule V drug and limited the amounts that can be purchased and requiring I.D. to purchase this substance.

Designer drugs are specifically made to fit around existing drug laws. A designer drug is a structural or functional analog of a controlled substance that has been designed to mimic the pharmacological effects of the original drug while at the same time, avoid being classified as illegal and/or avoid detection in standard drug tests. The most common designer drugs are created by making a derivative of an existing drug's chemical structure. This variation allows the drug to have similar effects as the illicit drugs, but the drugs will not fall under the drug laws. Designer drugs are usually variations on drugs that already exist.

These drugs, therefore, fall outside of the laws of the DEA. The variation of the chemical structure allows the drug to be created without the fear of any criminal charges because it is not under any current regulations.

## 10. Drug Abuse

Most drugs, especially pain medications may become ineffective if the medication is abused. Drugs are chemicals that have a profound impact on the neurochemical balance in your brain. This action affects how you feel and act. People who are suffering emotionally use drugs to escape from their problems. This can lead to drug abuse and addiction. Some physicians are afraid to prescribe scheduled drugs because of the possibility of causing addiction. Addiction is a chronic relapsing brain disease. Brain imaging shows that addiction severely alters your brain areas critical to decision-making, learning and memory, and behavior control, which may help to explain the compulsive and destructive behaviors of addiction. An addiction is a recurring problem by an individual to engage in some specific activity, despite harmful consequences to the individual's health, mental state or social life.

An addiction can occur with drugs, gambling, overeating, etc. Drugs can make you euphoric. As a result, you may request more and more drugs to maintain this euphoria. Drug abuse or substance abuse, involves the repeated and excessive use of prescription or street drugs. In one way or another, almost all drugs over stimulate the pleasure center of the brain, flooding it with the neurotransmitter dopamine which produces euphoria.

That heightened sense of pleasure can be so compelling that the brain wants that feeling back, again and again.

Addiction is frequently found in people with a wide variety of mental illnesses, including anxiety disorders, unipolar and bipolar depression, schizophrenia, and borderline and other personality disorders. Methadone can be used for the treatment of pain in addicted patients. Methadone is also an opiate that prevents users from getting high on heroin by competing with the much more potent opiates for the body's opiate receptors. Buprenorphine is another drug that is effective for the treatment of addiction and is also an analgesic.

Addiction and drug dependence occur when drugs become so important that you are willing to sacrifice your work, home and even your family. Once your brain and body get used to the substances you are taking, you begin to require increasingly larger and more frequent doses, in order to achieve the same effect.

Narcotics such as Heroin may over-stimulate the pleasure centers of the brain producing euphoric effects that cause compulsive drug-seeking behaviors. The severities of withdrawal symptoms associated with narcotics include chills, shakes, muscle pain, nausea, vomiting, and headaches and cravings.

A clinician must be able to distinguish between legitimate patients with chronic pain, and individuals engaged in nontherapeutic drug seeking behavior. Physicians have for years recognized the value of opioid analgesics in relieving chronic pain. Unfortunately, drug seekers may also request opioid analgesics. They do this by feigning illnesses, and seek controlled substances from multiple doctors and by forge prescriptions.

Drug seekers may be difficult to distinguish from true chronic pain sufferers. In general, drug seekers prefer illicit drugs such as heroin and cocaine to prescription drugs. Prescription drugs, however, have advantages over illicit drugs. Third-party insurers or welfare-entitlement programs may pay for prescribed drugs. Prescription pharmaceuticals are obtained in the safety of the physician's office.

Drug abuse and addiction have a devastating impact on society. Heroin use alone is responsible for the epidemic number of new cases of HIV/AIDS and hepatitis. Drug abuse is responsible for decreased job productivity and attendance, increased healthcare costs, and an escalation of domestic violence and violent crimes.

An estimated 20 percent of people in the United States have used prescription drugs for non-medical reasons. Central nervous stimulants, depressants and opioids are prescription drugs that are frequently abused. Central nervous system depressants are used to treat anxiety, panic attacks, and sleep disorders. Examples are Nembutal (pentobarbital sodium), Valium (diazepam), and Xanax (alprazolam). Long-term use can lead to physical dependence and addiction. Central nervous system stimulants are used to treat narcolepsy and the attention deficit/hyperactivity disorder. Examples include Ritalin (methylphenidate) and Dexedrine (dextroamphetamine). Opioids, also known as narcotic analgesics are used to treat pain. Opioids are the most commonly abused prescription drugs. Examples include morphine, codeine, OxyContin (oxycodone), Norco (hydrocodone) and Demerol (meperidine).

One may obtain drugs by the following means: prescription forgery, by telephone (faking to be a physician's office), multiple doctors, and indiscriminate prescribing by physicians. Pain clinicians who prescribe chronic opioids are aware that there is an illicit market for opioid analgesics. For example, OxyContin can be sold for $1.00 per milligram in some areas. One 80 mg pill can be sold on the street for $80.00. Telephone scams occur when the drug seeker claims to be a patient of one of the other physicians in the on-call group, and asks for a prescription for an analgesic to last until they can see their regular physician. Sometimes, the drug seeker uses a telephone to impersonate a practicing physician.

Prescription forgery is a common activity among drug seekers. Drug seekers can modify a legitimate prescription to increase the dosage or quantity of an opioid. The easiest method is to increase the number of tablets on the prescription. Multiple episodes of noncompliance raise an alert of drug seeking behavior as well as multiple episodes of prescription loss. The patient with chemical dependency loses control over drug taking. The patient cannot take medications as prescribed. The patient repeatedly reports lost or stolen medications.

The physician will notice that the drug seeker frequently requests early renewals of prescriptions. A pain physician must, however, be aware that aggressive complaining about the need for more drugs may indicate inadequate pain management as opposed to drug seeking behavior. A patient should not be allowed to suffer. It should be understood that substance abusers can suffer from chronic pain, which should be treated in a humane manner.

Unapproved use of opioids to treat another symptom such as sleep deprivation should not be tolerated. However, the pain management physician must objectively identify a patient's pain complaint with the appropriate medical test before prescribing an opioid. Opioids develop physical dependence and sometimes develop tolerance, but do not usually develop addictive disorders. Addiction is a primary chronic disease and exposure to opioid medications is only one of the etiologic factors in its development. Therefore, good clinical judgment must be used in determining whether the pattern of behaviors signals the presence of addiction or reflects a different issue.

Analgesics are powerful tools in the armamentarium of the pain clinician. Criminal and chemically dependent drug seekers may attempt to obtain such drugs from the physician.

A pain medicine physician must therefore, use safe prescribing strategies. A physician has no legal obligation to prescribe opioid analgesics on demand. A reasonable precaution to be taken by the pain medicine physician with an unfamiliar patient is to establish a policy of not prescribing opioid analgesics pending a complete assessment, including corroboration of the patient's history. Some patients or patient families are afraid of addiction. However, a significant number of individuals do not understand the difference between addiction and tolerance.

The American Academy of Pain Medicine, the American Pain Society, and the American Society of Addiction Medicine recognize the following definitions and recommend their use when discussing drug related behavorial problems.

I. Addiction

Addiction is a primary, chronic, neurobiological disease, with genetic, psychosocial, and environmental factors influencing its development and manifestations. It is characterized by behaviors that include one or more of the following: impaired control over drug use, compulsive use, continued use despite harm, and craving. An entity termed pseudo-addiction exists, which is not true addiction. Pseudo-addiction occurs when pain is under treated. Pseudo-addiction resolves when the pain addiction resolves. Addictive behavior on the other hand persists in spite of increasing the patient's pain medication.

II. Physical dependence

Physical dependence is a state of adaptation that is manifested by a drug class specific withdrawal syndrome that can be produced by abrupt cessation, rapid dose reduction, decreasing blood level of the drug, and/or administration of an antagonist.

III. Tolerance

Tolerance is a state of adaptation in which exposure to a drug induces changes that result in a diminution of one or more of the drug's effects over time. Most specialists in pain medicine and addiction medicine agree that patients treated with prolonged opioid therapy usually do develop physical dependence and sometimes develop tolerance, but do not usually develop addictive disorders. Addiction is a primary chronic disease and exposure to opioid medications is only one of the etiologic factors in its development. Therefore, good clinical judgment must be used in determining whether the pattern of behaviors signals the presence of addiction or reflects a different issue.

## 11. Drug Dosing

Does a one size dose fit all? Assume that you discovered a new plant that could treat hypertension. You want to put it in a pill and market it. How would you determine the dose of this drug to effectively treat the hypertension? A dose of medicine is the amount of medicine that should be taken at one time or regularly during a period of time in order to treat a medical condition. Determining the optimal dosage is an important step in the development of a drug.

The initial drug dose is recognized in a Phase I trial which was described in a previous chapter. In a Phase I trial, a small group of healthy volunteers is given the drug to see if it is safe how quickly it is absorbed, metabolized, and excreted from your body. In Phase II, a group of volunteer patients with the disease are given the drug to see how effective it is against the disease in question, what doses are most effective and what side effects occur. A control group of similar size is given a dummy drug which is called a placebo. The trials are blinded, which means that neither subjects nor the investigators know which pill a subject is receiving. In Phase III trials, thousands of patients with the disease are given the drug to get reliable data on its effectiveness, safety, therapeutic dose and side effects. The new drug is compared with the drugs that are currently used for treatment of the disease in question.

The drug manufacturer subsequently applies to the Food and Drug Administration for a new drug application. If it is granted, the generic name of the drug is replaced by a brand name chosen by the manufacturer. In Phase IV, the drug continues to be monitored to study if any unexpected side effects are reported. In the preclinical stage of drug development, an investigational drug must be tested extensively in the laboratory to ensure it will be safe to administer to humans. Testing at this stage can take up to five years and must provide information about the chemical composition of the drug, its safety and how the will be administered to the first human subjects. Pharmacological testing determines effects of the drug on the body. Toxicology studies are also conducted to identify potential risks to humans.

In the United States, the results of all animal drug testing must be provided to the U.S. Food and Drug Administration to obtain permission to begin clinical testing in humans. Regulatory agencies review the specific tests and documentation required to proceed to the next stage of development. Animal testing is used to measure how much of a drug is absorbed into the blood, how it is broken down chemically in the body, the toxicity of the drug and its breakdown products called metabolites, and how quickly the drug and its metabolites are excreted from the body.

A pharmacologic effect is exerted when the drug concentration at the site of action attains a minimum level. In many instances, the intensity of the pharmacologic effect is proportional to the drug concentration, with a greater effect attained at higher drug levels. However, there is an upper limit where a drug concentration triggers a maximal effect, and additional increases in drug concentrations do not promote a greater than a maximal effect. At this point, higher drug concentrations may lead to a variety of adverse effects, either due to too high of a drug level at the site of action and/or high drug levels exerting undesired effects at other organ and tissue sites of the body.

The onset of a pharmacological effect occurs when a minimum amount of drug distributes to the site of its pharmacologic action. The end of a pharmacological effect occurs when sufficient drug distributes away from the site of action. The amount of drug is then less than a minimum amount to elicit an effect.

Following drug administration, the absorbed drug dispenses into the bloodstream. The drug then distributes into various organs and tissues, including the site of pharmacologic action. When enough drug goes to the pharmacologic action site, a minimal effect is detected. As more drugs are distributed to the pharmacologic action site, a larger effect is witnessed. However, a drug in the bloodstream is also distributing into the liver and kidneys, which are working to eliminate the drug. Eventually, as the liver and kidneys eliminate more drug, the blood concentration of the drug decreases.

The drug in other organs and tissues, including the site of pharmacologic action, distributes out of the organs and tissues back into your bloodstream. In this manner, drug concentrations in the body continually decrease. Eventually, the amount of drug at the site of pharmacologic action reaches an amount just below the minimum amount to trigger an effect. At this point, the pharmacologic effect of the drug is terminated.

Studies on a new drug will evaluate the rate and extent to which the drug's active ingredient is made available to the body and the way it is distributed, metabolized, and eliminated from the body. Appropriate drug dosing is important for the drug safety and the efficacy of the new drug. This determination is primarily determined Phase II by means of dose-response studies.

Many factors must be considered with respect to the effect of drug action on your body. First, different drugs exert different effects on various body receptors, and unless a drug is able to exert an effect on some receptors, no reaction to the drug will take place. Other factors, such as the age, weight, gender, and genetics influence, can also affect the action of a drug.

The effect of a drug on the body depends upon its interaction with a particular body receptor and the function of that receptor in the body. In most cases, a drug must bond with the cell membrane in order for an action to take place. The point on the cell where the interaction takes place is called the receptor site. The specificity of the drug action among chemically related drugs usually depends upon the degree of fit between the drug and its receptor molecule. Drugs act on a receptor in the following ways: 1. Increase the activity of the receptor. 2. Decrease the activity of the receptor. 3. Block the activity of the receptor. In some cases, after a drug enters the body, it must be chemically altered before it is able to exert any effect at all on the body receptors.

The dose response of a particular drug differs for all drugs in the intensity and effects which is dependent on the dose of the drug given. Most drugs do not show an effect until a certain minimal level of dosage is reached. The smallest dosage of the drug to show an effect is the threshold of the drug. As the result of heredity, different people respond in a different manner to the same dosage of a drug. In most cases, the more of a drug one takes, the stronger effect of the drug.

The time that it takes for a drug to exert its desired effect once it has entered the body is important. Some drugs act immediately upon entering the circulatory system, and other drugs take hours and sometimes even days to exert their desired effects. Drugs that act immediately are designated short term and regularly require only single doses, whereas other drugs must be given in repeated dosages to be effective and are often called long-term effect drugs.

Many drug recommended dosages are for the average adult patient, as determined by clinical trials. The recommended dose is based on positive responses of the majority of patients with minimal or tolerable side effects. In many instances, the recommended drug dosage is appropriate for the majority of the average population. However, for some drugs, the prescribed dose may need to be individualized for patients suffering from other diseases that require other medications, advanced age, body weight, gender, etc. A one size dose does not fit all approach may be a reason why a drug does not always work in a patient.

Clinically effective drugs often have a therapeutic concentration range, whereby the minimum blood concentration is that concentration which causes a minimal pharmacologic effect. The maximum blood concentration is that concentration of drug that gives a maximum pharmacologic effect with no or minimal side effects. The therapeutic concentration range is determined by measuring the drug concentrations in a person's bloodstream and the intensity of the pharmacologic effect. Blood concentrations of a drug that are below the therapeutic range result in inadequate drug therapy. Blood drug concentrations within the therapeutic range lead to effective drug therapy. Blood drug concentrations that are above the therapeutic range frequently can cause harm.

On the other hand, when identical doses of a drug are given to individuals, large differences in pharmacologic responses may be seen. The dose required to produce a response may vary from individual to individual. Many factors contribute to the variability in the relationship between the administered dose and drug responses. Age, genetic factors, environmental factors, other diseases, and other drugs add to individual patient variability. Therapeutic drug monitoring may be performed whereby measurement of a person's blood drug concentrations provides guidance for drug dosage adjustment based on whether the blood concentrations are within or outside of the therapeutic range.

Be mindful that only a fraction of administered drug allocates to the tissue that is the site of the pharmacologic action. The drug is distributed to the liver, where it is metabolically changed into an inactive form in the process of metabolism. The drug is filtered into the urine by your kidneys in the process of elimination. At this time, insufficient drug is at the site of action to cause a pharmacologic effect. The quantity of drug that enters your bloodstream is determined by absorption processes. The amount of drug that arrives at the site of action is determined by the drug distribution process. Elimination of the drug is determined by the metabolism of the drug.

A pharmacologic effect is exerted when the drug concentration at the site of action attains a minimum level. In many instances, the intensity of the pharmacologic effect is proportional to the drug concentration. There is a higher limit where drug concentrations trigger a maximal effect, and additional increases in drug concentrations do not promote a greater result. At this point, higher drug concentrations may lead to a variety of adverse effects.

The therapeutic concentration range is determined by measuring the drug concentrations in a person's bloodstream and the intensity of the pharmacologic effect. Blood concentrations of drug that are below the therapeutic range frequently lead to inadequate control of the disease state. Blood drug concentrations within the therapeutic range lead to effective drug therapy. Blood drug concentrations that are above the therapeutic range may cause drug toxicities. For some drugs, when individuals are given identical doses of a drug, large differences in pharmacologic responses may be seen. Also, the dose required to elicit a desired response may vary widely from individual to individual.

Many factors contribute to the variability in the relationship between the administered dose and blood drug concentrations which indicates that one dose does not fit all patients.

## 12. Drug Effects in the Elderly

Older individuals are those who are over 65 years of age. Because of the baby-boomer generation, between the years 2010 and 2030, the population of the United States over 65 years of age will increase to 73%. One out of every five Americans will be over 65 years old. The majority of these individuals will require life time medical care. A problem exists in attempting to determine who will pay for this care.

Why do we age? Your body begins aging after you reach age 20. Body changes range from those affecting your cells throughout your body. As a result, aging affects s your joints, organs (i.e. heart, kidneys) brain, etc. Over time as you age, your cells lose the ability to repair themselves. Your cells in your body essentially wear out. Consequently, your joints become arthritic, your muscle mass decreases; your hair becomes thin, your bones fracture easily, etc. Your genetic makeup (DNA) determines when your body begins to wear out. In other words, your body is designed to wear out. Almost everyone experiences pain at some time, but elderly individuals experience the most pain. Their pain affects them emotionally. Elderly individuals who are unable to care for themselves have more pain than independent elderly patients. Depression is more common in the elderly population. Chronic pain can worsen an elderly patient's depression.

Liver size and liver blood flow decrease after age 50. Liver function can also be compromised in elderly patients. This decreased function can affect the breakdown of many drugs. As a result, the patient's blood level for a particular drug can be increased. This increase could cause drug toxicity which means that you may have too much drug in your body. You could die because of this. A younger patient usually has a greater body mass than an older individual. A dose of drug will be distributed through various body tissues. If you are emaciated, the dose of the drug will remain in your blood stream instead of being distributed throughout your body. As a result, the concentration of drug in your blood stream may be higher than expected. Decreased saliva noted in some older patients may interfere with swallowing. Drugs prescribed by mouth may be absorbed differently than younger persons because of changes in stomach acid levels in older patients.

Medication management in elderly patients can be a challenge. The reason is that physiologic changes occur in an elderly patient's bodies that include: the heart, lungs, kidneys, brain and sensation. If you are elderly, your heart rate may eventually decrease making it hard for your tissues to get oxygen while you exercise. Your lungs may not be able to ventilate like they did when you were younger. You may get short of breath when you exercise. Your kidneys become smaller with aging making it hard for you to excrete some drugs. Your liver size decreases, which can make it hard for you to metabolize some drugs. You can have decreased acid production in your stomach. This can cause a decrease in drug absorption from your stomach. In other words, when you take a medication, it may not be absorbed from your stomach into your blood. As a result, you will not derive any benefit from the medication. Your brain will shrink as well. Your ability to hear, smell and see will decrease as you age.

Elderly patients can be taking many different medications, prescribed by many physicians. Some of these drugs can adversely interact with some other medications and do not allow the current medication to be effective. Senile patients may forget to take their medications as prescribed. Their kidneys do not function as well as in younger patients. Your kidneys are responsible for eliminating drugs. As a result, drugs like morphine can accumulate within an elderly patient's body which could cause a drug overdose. Your liver metabolizes (breaks down drugs). Liver size and liver blood flow decrease after age 50.

Liver function can also be compromised in elderly patients. This decreased function can affect the breakdown of many drugs. As a result, the patient's blood level for a particular drug can be increased. As you age, your kidney function decreases. Your kidneys excrete drugs. If you cannot excrete a drug or it's by products, you could possibly be overdosed by the drug. Morphine by-products are excreted by your kidneys. If you have too much of a morphine break down product in your body, you may experience an overdose.

A younger patient usually has a larger total body muscle mass than an older individual. When he or she takes a medication, a portion goes to the muscles and other tissues. In other words, it temporarily leaves the blood stream. A dose of drug is supposed to be distributed throughout your various body tissues. If you are emaciated, a dose of drug will remain in your blood stream instead of being distributed throughout your body. As a result, the concentration of drug in your blood stream may be higher than expected. You may then experience an overdose of your medication. Drugs prescribed by mouth may be absorbed differently than younger persons because of changes in stomach acid levels in older patients. The changes in physiology associated with aging may increaser the side effects of many drugs.

Medications must be prescribed with prudence in elderly patients. Elderly patients can lose the ability for the stomach to repair itself, for example, after taking a drug that could cause ulcers (i.e. aspirin, ibuprofen, etc.). The goal of medication management is to decrease your symptoms so that you can maintain your normal activities of daily living. This means that your disease should not interfere with your family or recreation.

Medical and surgical treatments also contribute to pain in the elderly. It has been shown that older adults do not receive adequate pain management during hospitalization and commonly are given significantly fewer postoperative pain relievers than younger patients with the same diagnosis. This practice is particularly troublesome in light of research that demonstrates better patient outcomes, reduced length of stay, and reduced resource use as a result of aggressive pain control and improved mobility.

Medication management in elderly patients must be tailored to each patient needs with attention to each patient's overall medical condition. There must not be a "one size fits all" mentality when treating an elderly patient. It is your choice as to which pain management modalities or methods could work best for you with respect to your pain management.

## 13. Drugs in Pediatric Patients

Drug treatment in children differs from that in adults, most obviously because it is usually based on weight or surface area. Doses and dosing intervals differ because of age-related variations in drug absorption, distribution, metabolism, and elimination. A child cannot safely receive an adult drug dose, nor can it be assumed that a child's dose is proportional to an adult's dose. Most drugs have not been adequately studied in children.

For drugs, a child is defined as a person up to 17 years of age. If the product is to be used only for children, then it must be studied in the pediatric population. However, many therapies are developed for adults and then used in children without having been studied in children. Therefore, most marketed products that are mostly used in adults have not been studied in children even though they may be used by doctors to treat children.

As of 2008, an estimated 50 to 60 percent of prescription drugs used to treat children have been studied in some part of the pediatric population. Still, the likelihood that a medicine has actually been studied in neonates children less than a month old is close to zero. A common approach has been to use data from adults and adjust the dose according to a child's weight. Experimenting over the years has taught doctors to use many drugs in children safely and effectively. But this trial-and-error approach has also resulted in tragedy, indicating that adult experiences with a drug aren't always a reliable predictor of how children will react.

Most OTC products other than those for fever or pain have not actually been studied in children for effectiveness, safety, or dosing. They were approved for marketing many decades ago under a process where an expert panel looked at the evidence, including literature, and decided if a product should continue to be sold OTC. Most of the time, these panels did not have pediatric studies and were mostly using information collected in adults to determine if the product could be used in children.

There must be compelling reasons why a trial should be conducted in the pediatric population. Pediatric trials are in general more difficult to carry out because you must have special facilities, laboratory and radiological services, and staff that know how to work with children and their families. The high cost and difficulties associated with these trials are not attractive to sponsors who make these products.

Know that children can have different adverse reactions to a drug than adults. So for a product that has not been studied in children, it is possible for an adverse effect to occur that may not be listed on the drug's label. Children are more sensitive than adults to many drugs. For example, antihistamines and alcohol which are common ingredients in cold medications can have adverse effects at lower doses on young patients, causing excitability or excessive drowsiness. Some drugs, like aspirin, can cause serious illness or even death in children with chickenpox or flu symptoms.

A product is made up of many components. Some of these are inactive and only help make it taste better or dissolve better. Unless it is a combination product, usually there is only one active ingredient in a medication that causes the medicine to be effective against the disease or a condition. Many products, including products that treat different conditions, use the same active ingredients or the same class of active ingredients. For example, products to treat allergies may have the same active ingredient as some cough and cold products. So it is possible to overdose with a certain active ingredient if you are not careful.

The FDA recommends that OTC cough and cold medicines not be used to treat infants and children less than 2 years of age. Giving these products to these children can cause serious and potentially life-threatening side effects. The serious adverse events reported with cough and cold products include death, convulsions, rapid heart rates, and decreased levels of consciousness.

Both children and adults have different levels of enzymes in their livers for the processing drugs and these enzymes vary in concentration with age. This plays a vital role because certain drugs have to be tested specifically on children. Drug companies do not do these tests as they dislike the extra cost that has to be spent for these tests. But the companies and drug manufacturers have to keep this in mind when it comes to certain issues such as drug effectiveness and safety during early life stages. Remember that drug metabolism is the process by which the body breaks down and converts medication into active chemical substances.

They findings are very surprising because several of the enzymes vary in concentrations at different ages. One protein is the CYP3A4, which helps to metabolize some drugs in the body. It was found that children in the 2 year old age group have around 20-50 % of the CYP3A4 enzyme when compared to the adults. It is furthermore, frightening that 90 % of medicines used in the treatment of newborns were not tested on infants.

The very young and the very old often have limited liver function, which affects the ways in which the liver metabolizes drugs, resulting in lower thresholds for toxicity and unpredictable therapeutic effects. In the infant and young child, the liver has not yet fully developed and lacks the structural capacity to metabolize certain substances. Furthermore, many drugs do not undergo testing or evaluation for their effectiveness or safety in pediatric use because children make up a very small percentage of the drug's intended patient population or because the potential risks of involving children in clinical research studies are too high.

The continually changing metabolic capability and status of the child's body as organ systems grow and mature. The liver remains relatively unsophisticated in its function until a child reaches age 10 or 12 years. Not only does this limit the liver's ability to metabolize drugs such as antibiotics and pain medications, which are the most common kinds of drugs that children need, but also it makes the liver vulnerable to damage from substances that enter the blood circulation. Incompletely metabolized drugs increase the risk for damage to other developing organ systems as well.

Be aware that a wrong dosage of drug can cause a short-term toxicity or treatment failure in a pediatric patient. A child's physician must determine if a pediatric dose is within the safe dose range because of immature liver enzymes. When it comes to taking medicines, kids aren't just small adults. For prescription medicines, there is a pediatric section of the label. It says whether the medication has been studied for its effects on children. It also tells you what ages have been studied.

There are not many long term pediatric drug studies. This is unfortunate as these studies are necessary. An example of why long term studies are needed is a study from the Journal of the American Academy of Child and Adolescent Psychiatry which evaluated a stimulant drug, Ritalin that is used to treat ADHD. Ritalin did not improve children's symptoms long term. That may come as a surprise to parents, but ADHD researchers have been arguing for the past 10 years over the findings of the Multimodal Treatment Study of Children with ADHD.

This study is called the MTA study, it is the largest study conducted to compare the benefits of medication to behavioral interventions. This latest report from the MTA study tracked 485 children for eight years and found those still taking stimulant medication fared no better in the reduction of symptoms such as inattention and hyperactivity or in social functioning than those who hadn't. Most of the children who had taken medication for the first 14 months were no longer taking it. This, the researchers questioned about whether medication treatment beyond two years continues to be beneficial or needed at all.

The conclusion of the study was that stimulant drugs like Ritalin that are used to treat ADHD don't improve children's symptoms long term. This found those still taking stimulant medication fared no better in the reduction of symptoms such as inattention and hyperactivity or in social functioning than those who hadn't. Earlier reports found that children taking stimulants alone or combined with behavioral treatment did better in the first year than children who got no special care or who got behavioral treatment alone.

Furthermore, stimulant drugs stunt children's growth, according to another report in the journal that analyzes MTA data. Children who never took stimulants were three quarters of an inch taller and 6 pounds heavier on average than children who took medication for three years.

Important developmental changes in the gastrointestinal tract in children can occur that may affect oral absorption of medications. Developmental changes in the gastrointestinal tract with respect to medicines occur predominantly during the newborn period, infancy and early childhood. Consequently, drug doses will vary during this growth period as some drugs will be completely absorbed into a child's body while others may not. No information is available on effective and safe dosing regimens frequency of administration and duration of therapy of some drugs.

## 14. Drug Reactions

Severe drug interactions can occur when you take any medication. A drug interaction is a situation in which another drug or any substances, including food that can affect the activity of a drug that you are taking. The effects of the drug that you are taking may be increased or decreased. As previously mentioned in an earlier chapter, interactions between drugs occur which can cause drug-drug interactions. However, interactions may also exist between drugs & foods such as grapefruit juice, vegetables, fruits etc. These may occur out of accidental misuse or due to lack of knowledge about the ingredients involved in some substances.

A drug interaction, therefore, is an occurrence where a substance affects the activity of a drug when both are administered together. This action is synergistic when a drug's effect is increased or antagonistic when a drug's effect is decreased. Occasionally, a new effect can be produced by a drug that neither drug produces on its own.

Drug interactions may also occur between drugs and foods as well as other drugs and herbs. People taking some antidepressant drugs should not take food containing tyramine as an individual's blood pressure may become extremely elevated. A hypertensive crisis may occur. These interactions may occur to lack of knowledge about the ingredients involved in drugs or foods. Your pharmacist will warn you about potential serious drug interaction that is possible when you take a certain drug. Chocolate; alcoholic beverages, cheese, sour cream, yogurt, soy sauce, sauerkraut, beans, snow peas, bananas, pineapple, eggplants, figs, red plums, raspberries, nuts, and processed meats must be avoided when taking some antidepressants. Your prescribing physician and pharmacist will warn you about which foods to avoid with certain depression medications.

When an interaction between two drugs causes an increase in the effects of one or both of the drugs, this interaction is called a synergistic effect. Side effects are unwanted effects caused by the drugs. Most are mild, such as stomach aches or drowsiness, and go away after you stop taking the drug. Other effects can be more serious.

An adverse event is any undesirable experience associated with the use of a medical product in a patient. The event is serious and should be reported to FDA when the patient outcome is: death, life-threatening, hospitalization (initial or prolonged) required as a result of the drug. Disability or permanent damage must be reported if the adverse event resulted in a substantial disruption of a person's ability to conduct normal life functions. You should report an event to the FDA if you suspect that exposure to a medical product prior to conception or during pregnancy may have resulted in an adverse outcome in the child.

You must report an event when the current event does not fit the other outcome's criteria. An example is allergic bronchospasm, serious blood disorders or seizures that do not result in hospitalization. The development of drug dependence or drug abuse would also be examples of important adverse medical events.

Adverse drug reactions must therefore, be taken seriously. Adverse drug events (ADEs) are a serious public health problem. It is estimated that 82% of American adults take at least one medication. The rate of ADEs increases exponentially after a patient is on 4 or more medications. ADRs represent a significant public health problem that is, for the most part, preventable. It is estimated that 6.7% of hospitalized patients have a serious adverse drug reaction with a fatality rate of 0.32%.

Although some adverse drug reactions (ADR) are not very serious, others cause the death, hospitalization, or serious injury of more than 2 million people in the United States each year, including more than 100,000 fatalities. An adverse drug reaction is an injury caused by taking a medication. ADRs may occur following a single dose or prolonged administration of a drug or result from the combination of two or more drugs.

Adverse drug reactions are one of the leading causes of death in the United States. Furthermore, 750,000 people a year develop an adverse drug reaction after they are hospitalized. One third of adults in the United States take five or more medications. Elderly patients, who take more medications and are more vulnerable to specific medication adverse effects, are particularly vulnerable to ADEs. Children are also at elevated ADE risks as well.

Since older adults use significantly more prescription drugs than younger people, they have greatly increased odds of having a drug reaction caused by the dangerous interaction between two drugs. Often, older adults take one or more over-the-counter drugs in addition to their prescription drugs. This further increases the likelihood of adverse drug interactions. One of the more common kinds of adverse drug interactions is the ability of some drug to cause a second drug to accumulate to dangerous levels in the body.

To determine the cause of an ADR one needs to determine if the event was present before the patient began the medicine? Did the event occur within a plausible time period of starting the medicine? If a patient had the event prior to beginning the medication, then the medication did not cause the event. Sedatives and hypnotics were a leading source for adverse drug events seen in the hospital setting. The most common specifically identified causes of adverse drug events that originated during hospital stays were steroids, antibiotics, opiates and narcotics, and anticoagulants. More drugs are being used to treat patients than ever before. For example, 64% of all patient visits to physicians result in prescriptions. On the list of drugs most commonly identified in fatal events: oxycodone, fentanyl, morphine, acetaminophen, methadone, acetaminophen-hydrocodone and paroxetine. Drugs on the list of those most commonly identified in disability or serious outcomes include: estrogens, insulin, warfarin, atorvastatin, etanercept, simvastatin and venlafaxine. Approximately 2.8 billion prescriptions were filled in the year 2000. That is about 10 prescriptions for every person in the United States. Also, it is estimated that over 350,000 ADRs occur in U.S. nursing homes each year.

    The health care costs associated with adverse drug reactions is $136 billion annually which is more than the total cost of cardiovascular or diabetic care in the United States. Solutions to decrease ADR's include that the pharmacist must check for drug interactions and allergies, then release the appropriate quantity of the medication in the correct form. The correct medication must be supplied to the correct patient at the correct time. In the hospital medication dispensing is the nurse's responsibility, but in ambulatory care this is the responsibility of patients or caregivers.

## 15. Genetic Testing

Patients vary widely in their response to drugs. Genetic factors can account for 20 to 95 percent of patient variability. Drug therapy is ineffective in from 38% to 75% of therapeutic areas which could be remedied with genetic testing. For many drugs, there exist patients that are poor metabolizers (PM), intermediate metabolizers (IM), and ultrarapid metabolizers (UM). The risk of toxicity may increase for poor and intermediate metabolizers whereas for ultrapid metabolizers, these patients may require higher than normal doses for a therapeutic effect. The pharmaceutical industry has been focused on the blockbuster, a drug that can yield billions of dollars in revenue. The industry is concerned that it will not be able to maximize the patient base able to use a certain drug, and thereby revenue and profits, if it adopts genetic testing.

Genes in your cells provide your body with instructions for making enzymes. These enzymes are responsible for affecting how your medications work within your body. The study of genetic variations in drug response is called pharmacogenetics when studying an individual gene, or pharmacogenetics when studying all genes.

Pharmacogenetics is the study of the role of genetics in drug response. A person's genotype is his or her genetic makeup.

The term can pertain to all genes or to a specific gene. The phenotype is a person's outward physical appearance or function resulting from the interaction between the genotype and the environment. Genetic polymorphisms are naturally-occurring variants in gene structure that occur in more than 1 percent of the population. Polymorphisms may influence a drug's action by changing its pharmacokinetics or its pharmacodynamics. Enzymes are needed for your body to break down drugs so your body can get the benefit from the medicine. Differences in genes can affect the speed of action of different enzymes you have in your body. This affects how well your body can use medicines and how well drugs work in your body. Differences in your enzymes can affect how your body can break down a drug and how long the drug stays your body. Based on what type of genes you carry, you may be: a poor drug metabolizer, an extensive or "normal" drug metabolizer.

If you are a "poor metabolizer", you do not break down drugs well. This may result in too many drugs in the body which may lead to a dangerous side effect or even death. In some cases, your body may not be able to break down certain drugs to their working form and therefore, the drugs will not work properly. You metabolize drugs at the normal rate if you are an extensive or "normal" drug metabolizer. In other words, you metabolize drugs at a normal rate. If you are an "ultra-rapid" metabolizer, this means you break down drugs too fast, causing them to be of no use in the body. If medications do not work properly, conditions such as high blood pressure, blood disorders, and cancer will be left untreated and may even lead to death.

Your doctor will adjust the dose of your medication so that it is the correct right dose for you. Poor metabolizers might need to take a lower dose because they break down drugs slowly. Ultra-rapid metabolizers might need a higher dose because they break down drugs too fast.

Research shows that genetic factors account for a substantial proportion of all elements contributing to a patient's response to drugs in addition to age, sex, weight and liver function.

Genes provide your body with instructions for making enzymes, which help break down drugs in your system, allowing your body to benefit from the medicine that you take. Differences in your enzymes can affect how your body metabolizes a drug and how long the drug stays your body.

The most prevalent drug-metabolizing enzymes are the Cytochrome P450 enzymes. The human Cytochrome P450 family consists of 57 genes, with 18 families and 44 subfamilies. Cytochrome P450 proteins are conveniently arranged into these families and subfamilies based on similarities identified between amino acid sequences. Enzymes that share 35-40% identity are assigned to the same family by an Arabic numeral, and those that share 55-70% make up a particular subfamily with a designated letter.[18] For example, CYP2D6 refers to family 2, subfamily D, and gene number 6.

From a clinical perspective, the most commonly tested Cytochrome P450 enzymes include: CYP2D6, CYP2C19, CYP2C9, CYP3A4 and CYP3A5. These genes account for the metabolism of approximately 80-90% of current prescription drugs.

Enzymes produced from the cytochrome P450 genes are involved in the formation and breakdown of various molecules and chemicals within cells. Cytochrome P450 enzymes play a role in the synthesis of many molecules, including steroid hormones, cholesterol and other fatty acids, and acids used to digest fats. Additional cytochrome P450 enzymes metabolize external substances, such as medications that are ingested and internal substances, such as toxins that are formed within cells. There are approximately 60 cytochrome P450 genes in humans.

Cytochrome P450 enzymes are primarily found in liver cells but are also located in cells throughout the body. Within cells, cytochrome P450 enzymes are located in a structure involved in protein processing and transport and the energy-producing centers of cells. The enzymes found in the inner aspects of cells (mitochondria) are generally involved in the synthesis and metabolism of internal substances, while enzymes in the outer part of the cell (endoplasmic reticulum) usually metabolize external substances, primarily medications and environmental pollutants.

Common variations (polymorphisms) in cytochrome P450 genes can affect the function of the enzymes. The effects of polymorphisms are most prominently seen in the breakdown of medications. Depending on the gene and the polymorphism, drugs can be metabolized quickly or slowly. If a cytochrome P450 enzyme metabolizes a drug slowly, the drug stays active longer and less is needed to get the desired effect. A drug that is quickly metabolized is broken down sooner, and a higher dose might be needed to be effective. Cytochrome P450 enzymes account for 70 percent to 80 percent of enzymes involved in drug metabolism.

Each cytochrome P450 gene is named with CYP, indicating that it is part of the cytochrome P450 gene family. The gene is also given a number associated with a specific group within the gene family, a letter representing the gene's subfamily, and a number assigned to the exact gene within the subfamily. For example, the cytochrome P450 gene that is in group 26, subfamily B, gene 2 is written as CYP26B2.

Diseases caused by mutations in cytochrome P450 genes typically involve the buildup of substances in the body that are harmful in large amounts or that prevent other necessary molecules from being produced.

Common pain medications require activation by an enzyme called CYP2D6 to become effective. Approximately half of patients have genes that alter the function of CYP2D6. Testing for these gene alterations allows for changes to dosage regimens in order to compensate for altered metabolisms and can optimize the efficacy of your pain medication.

Ultra-rapid metabolizers break down medications rapidly. Individuals who frequently need more doses of medication in order to relieve pain may be ultra-rapid metabolizers. Poor metabolizers, on the other hand, tend to have severe side effects at low doses.

Cytochrome P450 is a family of enzymes involved in the rate and extent of drug metabolism. Some patients being treated with pain medication, for example, may not experience expected pain relief if they are ultra-rapid or poor metabolizers. Cytochrome P450 may also be inhibited or induced by drugs, resulting in drug-drug interactions and leading to unanticipated, adverse drug reactions.

Patients can exhibit inconsistent responses to drug therapies, which are influenced by variations in DNA coding of the

Cytochrome P450 enzyme family. These enzymes affect the extent of drug metabolism, and understanding patient metabolism rate can help physicians determine accurate dosage of proper pain management medication. Identifying CYP450 polymorphisms in 2D6, 2C19, 3A4 and 3A5 will indicate the rate at which patients can be expected to metabolize a drug. These tests can classify a patient as an ultra-rapid metabolizer, extensive metabolizer, intermediate metabolizer or poor metabolizer.

Variations in this gene can cause a person to metabolize drugs more quickly or slowly than normal, or Cytochrome P450 Cytochrome P450 Cytochrome P450 not at all. These differences in drug metabolism can lead to potential drug interactions, overdosing, or under dosing.

More than 85% of patients have significant genetic variations in the most important cytochromes: CYP2D6, CYP2C9, CYP2C19, CYP3A4 and CYP3A5. For example, CYP3A4 and CYP3A5 affect the metabolism of one-half of the drugs in clinical use.

Patients who are poor metabolizers may have an increased risk of drug-induced side effects, or may experience inadequate pain relief. Patients characterized as poor metabolizers or ultra-rapid metabolizers may need adjustments in dosage depending on the drug. Cytochrome P450 test results may help develop a treatment strategy for patients using some medications.

If your medicine does not work, ask your physician if genetic testing is appropriate for you to help determine why your medication does not work. Pharmacogenetic testing may enable physicians to understand why patients react differently to various drugs and to make better decisions about therapy. Pharmacogenetics is a field that deals with the relationship between genetic variations and the effects and side-effects of drugs. Genetic variations in drug-metabolizing enzymes, transporters, receptors, and other drug targets have been linked to individual differences in the efficacy and safety of many drugs.

## 16. Anti-Inflammatory Drugs

Nonsteroidal anti-inflammatory drugs (NSAIDs) are drugs that provide pain-killing and fever reducing effects, as well as anti-inflammatory effects. Nonsteroidal anti-inflammatory drugs and may be recommended to help treat symptoms of headaches, sprains, arthritis, period pain, fever and swelling. Although NSAIDs can be very effective, there is a risk of side-effects including indigestion, ulcers, allergic reactions and heart problems. These drugs, however, do not decrease all types of pain. Pain can be defined as nociceptive when it is generated by noxious stimuli, (surgical wound, which responds to hydrocodone or equivalent medicine), inflammatory when produced by tissue injury and/or immune cell activation (which respond to NSAIDs), and neuropathic, when it is due to a lesion of the nervous system (which responds to anticonvulsant medications).

NSAIDs will primarily alleviate inflammatory pain by decreasing inflammatory prostaglandins. In the peripheral nervous system, NSAIDs work by decreasing the sensitivity of the nociceptor to painful stimuli. NSAIDs block the increased transmission of repetitive incoming signals from injured nerves to higher centers in your brain where pain is perceived. NSAIDs are more than just pain relievers. They also help reduce inflammation and lower fevers. They prevent blood from clotting, which is good in some cases but not so beneficial in others.

NSAIDs reduce the blood flow to the kidneys, which makes them work more slowly. When your kidneys are not working well, fluid builds up in your body. The more fluid in your bloodstream, the higher is your blood pressure. If you take NSAIDs in high doses, the reduced body blood flow can permanently damage your kidneys because your kidneys do not receive enough blood flow.

NSAIDs are usually indicated in the treatment of acute or chronic conditions where pain and inflammation are present. Nonsteroidal anti-inflammatory drugs are powerful analgesics, especially for nociceptive pain. NSAIDs also are effective in some neuropathic pain syndromes when used with other analgesics.

Prostaglandins are chemicals produced by the cells throughout your body and cause inflammation and also cause pain and fever; support the blood clotting function of platelets; and protect the lining of the stomach from developing ulcers. Prostaglandins are produced by the enzyme cyclooxygenase (COX). There are two COX enzymes, COX-1 and COX-2. Both enzymes produce prostaglandins that promote inflammation, pain, and fever. COX-1 protects the stomach.

Long-term use of NSAIDs has been associated with kidney failure, stomach ulcers and bleeding, and hypertension. The more an NSAID blocks Cox-1, the greater is its tendency to cause ulcers and bleeding. One NSAID called Celebrex, blocks Cox-2, but has a little effect on Cox-1. This drug is referred to as one of the selective Cox-2 inhibitors and therefore, causes less bleeding as and fewer ulcers than other NSAIDs. NSAIDs reduce the blood flow to your kidneys. Kidneys excrete body fluid. NSAIDs in high doses can reduce blood flow and can permanently damage your kidneys, which may cause kidney failure. Cox-2 inhibitors have been linked to an increased risk of heart attacks and strokes.

The Federal Drug Administration stated that patients who are at a high risk of gastrointestinal bleeding, have a history of intolerance to non-selective NSAIDs, or are not doing well on non-selective NSAIDs may be appropriate candidates for COX-2 selective agents. NSAIDs are classified as non-opioid analgesic drugs and are aspirin like drugs. Although the pharmacologic and toxicological properties of these compounds are similar and all possess analgesic activity, only certain drugs are indicated specifically for the relief of pain (e.g. Feldene, Voltaren, Advil, Naprosyn, and Celebrex).

All of the NSAIDs analgesics prevent the biosynthesis and release of prostaglandins by inhibition of prostaglandin cyclooxygenase, a cell membrane enzyme that is present in almost all cells. Therefore, the NSAIDs reduce the formation of prostaglandins and decrease the pain sensitivity caused by these substances.

Not all the drugs are equally active, nor are all clinically useful, with respect to their effects. Diflunisal, for example, is used exclusively as an analgesic but does not decrease a fever. Except for acetaminophen, aspirin, and ibuprofen, none of the other compounds are used to reduce fever. NSAIDS are used for the treatment of various arthritic conditions such as rheumatoid arthritis, ankylosing spondylitis, osteoarthritis and acute gouty arthritis. As the particular inflammatory condition being treated is alleviated, the pain associated with the disease is usually also decreased. Pain associated with inflammatory disease is effectively reduced by all NSAID drugs. The anti-inflammatory activity of NSADs in descending order is as follows: indomethacin > diclofenac > piroxicam > ketoprofen > lornoxicam > ibuprofen > ketorolac > acetylsalicylic acid.

Toradol (ketorolac) has minimal anti-inflammatory effects but has significant pain relieving effects and is used in many emergency departments for pain relief. This observation suggests that anti-inflammatory effects are not exclusively related to pain relieving effects.

Gastrointestinal toxicity can occur with all NSAIDS that can cause bleeding from the stomach and may lead to hospitalization and surgery as well as blood transfusions. Localized irritation of the stomach lining constitutes the most common adverse reaction associated NSAIDS. Although epigastric distress is common at the lower doses, gastric and/or intestinal ulceration and bleeding will occur in only a small percentage of patients. At higher doses of aspirin, erosive gastritis and gastrointestinal hemorrhage are observed more often. These effects are the result from the inhibition of cyclooxygenase 1 (COX-1).

You need cyclooxygenase-1 to form protective prostaglandins that reduce acid secretion by your stomach and promote the secretion of protective intestinal mucus. Aspirin and other compounds with high anti-inflammatory activity, such as indomethacin, tend to elicit the highest incidence of gastrointestinal reactions. Other NSAIDS like naproxen are considered to produce fewer and fewer intense gastrointestinal reactions than aspirin.

Acetaminophen is essentially devoid of these effects. Acetaminophen has some anti-inflammatory effects. Newer NSAIDS that are specific for cyclooxygenase 2 enzymes are safer than the rest of the NSAIDS that inhibit both cyclooxygenase 1 and 2. Celebrex is safer on your stomach. With respect to the heart and lungs all the NSAIDS can increase your blood pressure.

It should be noted that all NSAIDS could be linked to an increased risk of a heart attack. Because of this evidence, it is advisable to use the lowest effective dose of NSAID for the shortest time necessary. NSAIDS can also cause clotting problems and make you prone to bleeding or bruising. This is due to the inhibition of thromboxane A, formation in thrombocytes (cells in the bloodstream associated with clotting). However, Celebrex does not cause this problem. In other words, Celebrex is the only NSAID that does not adversely affect the blood-thinning effects of aspirin.

With respect to your kidneys, sodium and water retention with arms and legs, swelling is seen with NSAID use. The higher the dose, the more prone you are for these side effects. If you are over sixty years of age, you should be prescribed lower doses, as you may be more sensitive to NSAIDS than younger patients. NSAIDS are excellent analgesic medications for pain in extremities, as well as for dental pain and headaches. They are furthermore, non-addicting. An NSAID can adversely affect your kidneys. In some instances, NSAIDS can cause kidney failure.

NSAIDS should be used with caution in elderly patients. Nonsteroidal anti-inflammatory drugs (NSAIDs) are commonly used in the elderly for the treatment of fever, pain, pain associated with inflammation in rheumatoid arthritis and osteoarthritis, neuromuscular disorders, headache, and musculoskeletal conditions. Each year in the United States, people spend 5 to 10 billion dollars to purchase prescription and over-the-counter NSAIDs. Gastrointestinal side effects such as ulcers and bleeding are the most prevalent and life-threatening problems associated with NSAIDs in elderly individuals.

Specifically in the elderly, NSAIDs have become a leading cause of hospitalization in this age group and may increase the risk of death from ulceration more than four fold. NSAIDs and the new class of cyclo-oxygenase-2 selective NSAIDs continue as drugs of choice for analgesia and anti-inflammatory effects. Physiological changes of aging worsen the side-effect profile of NSAIDs in the elderly. These side effects, when added to the increased potential for drug interactions, lead to a much greater risk for adverse outcomes when NSAIDs are used in the elderly patient.

NSAIDS should be used with caution in pregnant patients as well. These drugs are not recommended during pregnancy, especially in the third trimester. While NSAIDs as a class are not direct congenital malformation drugs, they may, however, cause premature closure of the fetal ductus arteriosus and also cause a reduction in maternal amniotic fluid. As a result, pregnant patients taking NSAIDS may require ultrasound monitoring by the treating obstetrician. In addition, NSAIDS may cause premature birth. Aspirin should not be used during pregnancy. Fetal bleeding could occur as a result of the inhibitory effects on the fetal platelets. Acetaminophen which does have slight anti-inflammatory properties is safe and well-tolerated during pregnancy.

There are many different types of NSAIDs, which are categorized according to their chemical structures: Salicylates :( aspirin, salsalate), Pyrroles (ketorolac), COX-2 Inhibitors: (celecoxib), Arylalkanoic acids: ibuprofen, ketoprofen, naproxen, fenoprofen, flurbiprofen and oxaprozin pyrroles: ketorolac, Enolic acids (oxicams): piroxicam, meloxicam.

NSAIDs that inhibit both COX-1 and COX-2 enzymes are named non-selective NSAIDs. NSAIDs that mainly inhibit COX-2 enzymes are named COX-2 inhibitors. The following NSAIDs have pronounced selectivity towards COX-1 enzymes: aspirin, indomethacin. ketoprofen, piroxicam, and sulindac. Moderate selectivity towards COX-1 is noted with: diclofenac, iIbuprofen, naproxen. Equal inhibition of COX-1 and COX-2 include: etodolac, meloxicam, nimesulide, nabumetone. Pronounced selectivity towards COX-2: includes celecoxib.

Uricosurics act by increasing uric acid excretion in urine and are used for the treatment of gouty arthritis.. The primary goal in using uricosurics is to prevent or control the frequency of gouty arthritis attacks. Uricosurics are absorbed from the GI tract. Probenecid and sulfinpyrazone are indicated for the treatment of chronic gouty arthritis. Allopurinol is used to reduce production of uric acid, preventing gouty attacks, and colchicine is used to treat acute gouty attacks. Colchicine doesn't interact significantly with other drugs. When allopurinol is used with other drugs, the resulting interactions can be serious as allopurinol potentiates the effect of oral anticoagulants.

Numerous NSAIDs are available as generic drugs and include: diclofenac, etodolac, fenoprofen, flurbiprofen, ibuprofen, indomethacin, ketoprofen, meclofenamate, naproxen, piroxicam, sulindac, and tolmetin. Only meloxicam, nabumetone and oxaprozin are available by brand name only.

Remember, effective pain relief is not easy to achieve. If you suffer chronic pain, you may want to get a referral to a pain specialist. Furthermore, it's important to keep in mind that some pain can't be completely taken away.

Sometimes, being absolutely pain free from joint pain is simply not a realistic goal, but if you work with your doctor, you could at least try to get to the point where pain doesn't interfere with your daily life. Frequent or regular use of ibuprofen (an NSAID) may reduce the effectiveness of aspirin if you are taking it to prevent heart attacks or strokes. In addition, combining these medications may increase your risk of developing gastrointestinal ulcers and bleeding. You may need a dose adjustment or more frequent monitoring by your doctor to safely use both medications.

There are different classes of NSAIDS: If a medication in one class does not work, a medication from another class may provide you with relief. 1. Propionic acids: fenoprofen, flurbiprofen, ibuprofen, ketoprofen, naproxen and oxaprozin. 2. Acetic acids: diclofenac, indomethacin, sulindac and tolmetin. 3. Enolic acids: meloxicam and piroxicam. 4. Fenamic acids: meclofenamate and mefenamic acid. 5. Napthylalkanones: nabumetone. 6. Pyranocarboxylic acids: etodalac. 7. Pyrroles: ketorolac. 8. COX-2 inhibitors: celecoxib.

Your medications may not decrease your pain if you also suffer from nerve pain.

Using ibuprofen together with ketorolac can cause nausea, vomiting, stomach pain, drowsiness, black or bloody stools, coughing up blood, urinating less than usual, and shallow breathing. Do not use any other over-the-counter cold, allergy, or pain medication without first asking your doctor or pharmacist. Serotonin reuptake inhibitors (SRIs) may potentiate the risk of bleeding in patients treated with ulcerogenic agents and agents that affect hemostasis such as anticoagulants, platelet inhibitors, thrombin inhibitors, thrombolytic agents, or agents that commonly cause thrombocytopenia. The tricyclic antidepressant, clomipramine, is also a strong SRI and may interact similarly. Serotonin release by platelets plays an important role in hemostasis, thus SRIs may alter platelet function and induce bleeding. Published case reports have documented the occurrence of bleeding episodes in patients treated with psychotropic agents that interfere with serotonin reuptake. Bleeding events related to SRIs have ranged from ecchymosis, hematoma, epistaxis, and petechiae to life-threatening hemorrhages. Additional studies have confirmed the association between use of these agents and the occurrence of upper gastrointestinal bleeding, and concurrent use of NSAIDs or aspirin was found to potentiate the risk. Preliminary data also suggest that there may be a pharmacodynamic interaction between SSRIs and oral anticoagulants that can cause increased bleeding.

Only take NSAIDS with methotrexate or other arthritis specific medications. Ibuprofen, for example, may increase the blood levels and side effects of methotrexate. You may be more likely to experience this interaction if you have kidney disease or are receiving a high dose of methotrexate. The risk may be less if you are using methotrexate once a week to treat certain forms of arthritis.

Nonsteroidal anti-inflammatory agents can raise blood pressure in some people. Some people with known high blood pressure (hypertension) may have to stop taking NSAIDs, if they notice their blood pressure increases in spite of taking their blood pressure medications and following their diet. If you are taking antihypertension medication consult your health care provider before taking NSAIDs.

In general, medications may not work for the following reasons:

1. Most drugs are manufactured for a specific ailment. If your diagnosis is wrong, and if you were prescribed a specific drug for a disease, you will not receive any relief.

2. Your prescribed drug may be adversely affected by your hormones.

3. Other drugs that you are taking may interfere with your medicine. Drug-drug interactions occur when two or more drugs react with each other. Drug-food/beverage interactions result from drugs reacting with foods or beverages. Drug-condition interactions may occur when an existing medical condition makes certain drugs potentially harmful

4. Your drug won't work if it is not absorbed by your stomach or small intestine due to excess acid in your gut.

5. Many drugs will not work unless the drug is converted into a new medication in your liver. You may have a genetic mutation which prevents this conversion.

6. Your dose of medication may not be sufficient.

7. Your medicine may not be potent enough.

8. Most drugs need to be absorbed from your stomach or small intestine to enter your blood stream. Abdominal surgery may not leave a way for a drug to get into your blood stream.

9. Your liver may filter a large portion of the drug before it gets to the proper receptor.

10. Your kidneys may excrete your drug too quickly before it has time to give you relief.

11. Some foods that you eat may interact with your medication causing your medication not to work.

12. Smoking may inhibit the effects of some medications.

13. Many medications are divided into subclasses. A change from one subclass to another subclass may be effective for your condition.

14. Other factors can affect how quickly a drug is absorbed. For example, most absorption of oral drugs occurs in the small intestine. If a patient has had large sections of the small intestine surgically removed, drug absorption decreases. If your body does not absorb enough drug, it may not work.

15. Pain and stress can also decrease the amount of drug absorbed by your body.

16. Drug tolerance occurs when a patient develops a decreased response to a drug over time. You then require a larger dose of medication to produce the same response.

17. Some generic drugs may not work as well as the brand name drugs.

18. Your gender may affect how your drug works.

19. Medications may be given by mouth, by patch, by suppository, by injection or by nasal spray. If one form of drug is ineffective another form may work.

20. Some drugs compete for the same receptor (e.g. Narcan and Morphine where Narcan pushes the Morphine off the mu receptor which stops the effects of the Morphine).

21. You must read all the instructions and warnings that come with your medication for your drug to work effectively.

If your anti-inflammatory medication does not work, the drug may not be strong enough. The anti-inflammatory activity of NSADs in descending order as mentioned previously is as follows: indomethacin > diclofenac > piroxicam > ketoprofen > lornoxicam > ibuprofen > ketorolac > acetylsalicylic acid. You may need to take a stronger medication.

Serum urate levels may increase when probenecid is taken with antineoplastic drugs and make probenecid ineffective.

# WHY WON'T MY MEDICATION WORK?

## 17. Pain Medications

Another medical specialty, Pain Management, has emerged in recent years that treat patients with all varieties of chronic pain, often without a specific diagnosis. Narcotic drugs are prescribed for postoperative pain, cancer pain and for some chronic pain syndromes. Narcotic drugs can relieve moderate to severe pain. The term narcotic refers to agents that benumb or deaden nerves, causing loss of feeling or paralysis.

Psychedelic drugs like LSD are not narcotics. Many law enforcement officials in the United States inaccurately use the word "narcotic" to refer to any illegal drug or any unlawfully possessed drug. Physicians now prescribe addictive and powerful narcotics routinely to patients with a variety of chronic painful conditions. Over time, the patient becomes tolerant and addicted to these medicines. In many instances, the narcotic dependence and addiction become a much more serious disease than the original illness. We all know that opioid narcotics are highly addictive and come with severe adverse effects. They cause profound suppression of the endocrine system. Another adverse effect of long-term opioid use is opioid-induced hyperalgesia. This is a form of hypersensitivity to pain. The original painful condition becomes worse. Other adverse effects include impaired cognitive function, and suppression of the immune system.

Opioids are used for chronic pain management. Chronic pain is a progressive disease of the nervous system, caused by failure of the body's internal pain control systems. The disease is accompanied by changes in the biochemical and anatomical makeup of the spinal cord.

Acetaminophen is a drug that produces analgesic and antipyretic effects. It appears in many products designed to relieve moderate pain, including narcotic drugs. If you have severe pain acetaminophen may not be effective taken alone.

Many medical professionals prefer the term opioid which refers to natural, semi-synthetic and synthetic substances that behave pharmacologically like morphine. The Opioids are a class of controlled pain-management drugs that contain natural or synthetic chemicals based on morphine, the active component of opium. These narcotics effectively mimic the pain-relieving chemicals that the body produces naturally. Opioids are the most often prescribed pain-relievers because they are so effective. However, more than 16,600 people a year die from overdoses of the drugs, including methadone, morphine, and oxycodone and hydrocodone combined with acetaminophen. For every death, more than 30 other patients are admitted to the emergency room.

Opioid drugs work very well to alleviate severe short-term pain due to, say, surgery or a broken bone. They can also help with pain associated with terminal or very serious illnesses.

Some people do find that high doses take the edge off their pain, but the nausea, constipation, and fuzzy-headedness that commonly result from taking strong doses of an opioid make it not worth the benefit.

Some opioid analgesics, called mixed opioid agonist-antagonists, have agonist and antagonist properties. The agonist component relieves pain, while the antagonist component decreases the risk of toxicity and drug dependence. Morphine is the standard to which other opioid drugs are compared. Morphine is frequently prescribed to alleviate severe pain after surgery. Codeine can be helpful in soothing somewhat milder pain, as are oxycodone, hydrocodone, hydromorphone and meperidine, which is used less often because of its side effects. Diphenoxylate or lomotil can also relieve severe diarrhea, and codeine can ease severe coughs. Other drugs include oxymorphone and fentanyl. The mixed opioid agonist-antagonists include: buprenorphine (Buprinex patch), butorphanol (Stadol nasal spray) nalbuphine (Nubain) intravenous) and pentazocine (Talwin).

The principal use of opioids is to relieve pain. Other medical uses include control of coughs and diarrhea, and the treatment of addiction to other opioids. Opioids can produce euphoria, making them prone to abuse. Opioids should only be used for moderate to severe pain that has not responded to non-narcotic drugs like aspirin or ibuprofen.

Narcotics can be used alone like oxycodone or used in combination with aspirin, ibuprofen or acetaminophen. Some narcotics like oxycodone or morphine are available as an extended release tablet that must be swallowed whole. Tablets, which are not extended release, may be split.

There is a difference between the descriptions of narcotic drugs and opioids. Opioids are drugs like morphine, hydrocodone, etc. Narcotics are sometimes referred to as extremely addictive drugs and include heroin and other drugs that can cause sedation. Opioids act by attaching to a group of proteins called opioid receptors, found in the brain, spinal cord and gastrointestinal tract. When these drugs link to certain opioid receptors in the brain and spinal cord, they can block the transmission of pain messages to the brain.

For the purposes of discussion in outlining the pharmacologic activity of these compounds, the opioids will be classified as (1) agonists, (2) antagonists, and (3) mixed agonist-antagonists. All drugs bind to receptors that exist on the outer membrane of your cells. Narcotics bind to narcotic receptors on cells in the brain and spinal cord. Opioid receptors may also be recruited on tissue cells outside of your central nervous system such as your knee following an injury. An injection of morphine into your knee may alleviate your pain.

When opioids turn on a receptor, that receptor decreases pain signals usually in your spinal cord that prevents pain signals from going to your brain. As a result, your pain perception is decreased. Experimental studies involving binding of opioids to specific receptors in the brain and spinal cord have substantiated the hypothesis that these receptors exist, which mediates the actions of the opioid drugs to stop pain signals to your brain. There are two basic classes of opioid receptors called mu and kappa receptors. Kappa receptor stimulation can decrease your pain and causes less addiction potential.

Experimental evidence suggests that activation of mu receptors (found principally at sites in the brain) is associated with analgesia, respiratory depression, euphoria, and physical dependence. The kappa receptors (located within the spinal cord) are believed to mediate spinal analgesia, constriction of the pupil size and sedation. The other receptors may influence affective behavior, and although some physicians believe that activation of these receptors plays a role in opioid-induced analgesia; this remains controversial.

Agonistic opioids act as analgesics by binding to and activating both mu and kappa receptors in the brain and spinal cord. The opioid antagonists bind to all categories of opioid receptor sites throughout the body, but fail to activate them. These compounds are not used for pain control; rather, the utility of these drugs lies in their ability to reverse an overdose of opioids, including narcotics.

The compounds that comprise the mixed agonist-antagonist group are more recent additions to the clinically important opioids. These drugs are semi-synthetic derivatives of morphine, the chemical structures of which have agonistic activity at some kappa receptors but opposed activity at mu receptors, e.g., pentazocine, butorphanol, and nalbuphine, or partial agonistic activity at mu receptors and antagonistic activity at kappa receptors, eg. buprenorphine. All are effective analgesics since they stimulate either mu or kappa receptors.

Chemically, the opioid agonists include a number of classes of drugs, all of which have pharmacologic effects similar to those of morphine. Morphine is the oldest known drug of this class. It remains as the prototype for the opioid group and is the standard to which every other opioid analgesic drug is compared. Opioid drugs decrease pain but also affect all organ systems. Your pituitary gland in your brain can be adversely affected by chronic narcotic use. For example, in males opioids can decrease testosterone that can cause depression and erectile dysfunction. Drowsiness and blurred vision can occur. Changes in mood can occur. An inability to concentrate can occur.

Euphoria can be experienced in 20% of individuals taking opioid drugs. Euphoria can be the cause of addiction. Opioids can stop your respiratory drive that can cause you to stop breathing. Narcotics affect your stomach by slowing down the passage of food in combination with your brain to cause nausea and vomiting. Opioids can cause a significant decrease in your blood pressure that may cause you to fall. Opioids decrease movement of the bowel resulting in constipation. Morphine can make gall bladder disease worse by contracting a valve where the gall bladder meets the intestine called the sphincter of Oddi. Opioid drugs can result in a release of histamine from certain cell in the body that can cause itching and a rash. As you can see opioid drugs can have side effects.

Tolerance, addiction and physical dependence can occur with opioid drugs. Tolerance occurs when it takes more of the drug to cause the same decrease in your pain. This is not addiction. Patients may find that they develop tolerance to opioid pain medications and may need to have their doses increased in order to be effective. Tolerance has not been shown to lead to drug addiction. Physical dependence is a condition that occurs when continued use of the drug is needed to prevent a withdrawal reaction. Steady use of opioids can result in tolerance to the drugs so that higher doses must be taken to achieve the same effects. Long-term use also can lead to physical dependence where the body adapts to the presence of the drug, and withdrawal symptoms occur if use is reduced abruptly.

Addiction is an intense craving for an opioid and is often associated with recreational use. Signs and symptoms of addiction include yawning, sweating, restlessness, irritability, anxiety, nasal discharge, tearing, dilated pupils, gooseflesh, tremors, loss of appetite, body aches, nausea and vomiting, fever and chills and an increase in heart rate and blood pressure. These symptoms may last 7-10 days. Minor symptoms can begin in 8-12 hours after the last dose of the opioid. The more severe symptoms like nausea and vomiting to begin 48-72 hours after the last dose of the drug. With respect to agonist drugs, morphine is the prototype. It can be administered by mouth, rectum or by injection into muscle or vein. Is is prepared in a capsule, tablet or a liquid. It is available by a rectal suppository as well. This route of administration is used for those patients who cannot swallow or are having severe vomiting.

Hydromorphone and oxymorphone also come in the form of rectal suppositories. The duration of action of opioids varies from drug to drug. Sustained-release morphine and oxycodone give a longer duration of action. Immediate release drugs provide a faster onset but have a shorter duration of action. Fentanyl, which is 75 times more potent than morphine is available in a patch and sucker, forms. The fentanyl patch is used for severe constant pain. The pain relief is continuous. The sucker, which only comes in a raspberry flavor, is used for severe cancer pain in instances where the severe pain fluctuates. Fentora is another oral form of fentanyl.

With respect to the fentanyl pain patch, the amount of drug released is controlled by small holes in a membrane in the patch. A larger hole permits the release of fentanyl into your body. The patches are available in different doses. The fentanyl is released for 48-72 hours. Patients with a fever can be at a risk for an overdose as the amount of fentanyl administered to your body can increase by 25% for every 30C increase in body temperature. The advantage of the patch is that patients do not have to take frequent pills during the night. The patch should be applied to a hairless surface.

Tramadol (Ultram) is an interesting drug and may be used for moderate to moderately severe pain. It has a low abuse potential. It is not a scheduled drug. It activates mu and kappa receptors. The side effects are minimal when compared to opioid drugs. Tramadol does not produce withdrawal symptoms like opioids. The advantage of tramadol over other drugs is that tramadol inhibits norepinephrine and serotonin brain reuptake and can therefore be effective for the treatment of fibromyalgia pain. These two substances in the brain and spinal cord decrease fibromyalgia pain. The opioid drugs do not have this effect.

Tramadol can cause nausea dizziness and headaches. Tramadol does not lower the heart rate or blood pressure. Tramadol provides pain relief similar to codeine and propoxyphene.

Naloxone and naltrexone are drugs that reverse the respiratory effects of opioids. Naltrexone can be given orally. The only time that these drugs are given is to treat opioid intoxication.

Butorphanol (Stadol) and pentazocine (Talwin) are called mixed agonist-antagonists drugs. These drugs show receptor selectivity, and these two drugs stimulate kappa receptors. These drugs have fewer opioid abuse tendencies than the agonist drugs. Opioids, on the other hand, work on both mu and kappa receptors. Strong opioids exist, which are usually reserved for cancer patients or other patients with severe pain.

Hydromorphone (Dilaudid) and levorphanol (Levo-Droman) are eight and five times more potent than morphine. Meperidine (Demerol) is an opioid that is weaker than morphine. It is used infrequently in pain management as it can cause tremors or seizures if used on a chronic basis. Methadone is a synthetic drug similar to morphine. The advantage of methadone for your pain management is that it does not cause euphoria. Methadone, however, can cause a heart conduction problem in your heart. Consequently, patients have died from heart problems after being prescribed methadone. Hydrocodone and oxycodone are two opioids used for moderate to moderately severe pain. These drugs are usually combined with aspirin and acetaminophen, which can potentiate the analgesic efficacy of these drugs. Tapentadol (Nucynta) is an opioid analgesic with a dual mode of action as an agonist of the mu receptor and as a norepinephrine reuptake inhibitor. It has an analgesic effect comparable to oxycodone.

Another clinical fact is that you need to know is that opioid drugs can actually cause you to experience increased pain. This observation is called opioid induced pain. Many physicians are unaware of this fact. In this situation, a reduction in your dose of your medicine or stopping it can actually decrease your pain. This phenomenon can also be seen in patents that have spinal morphine drug-delivery systems.

As one can see, there are many opioids that can be used for the management of your acute chronic pain. The proper choice of your medication is dependent on the magnitude of your pathology, the side effects of the drug prescribed, the effectiveness of the drug and your overall health.

Why won't my medications work?

Some pain medications are more potent than others as mentioned above. There are many types of analgesics. Your doctor may have to try more than one medication to find one that decreases your pain.

Opioid analgesics include the following: acetaminophen with codeine (Tylenol #2, #3, #4), buprenorphine (Butrans), fentanyl transdermal patches (Duragesic), hydrocodone with acetaminophen (Lortab Elixir, Vicodin), hydrocodone with ibuprofen (Vicoprofen), hydrocodone (Zohydro), hydromorphone (Exalgo), meperidine (Demerol, Merpergan), methadone (Dolophine), morphine and morphine sustained release (MS-Contin, Avinza, Kadian), oxycodone sustained release (OxyContin), oxycodone with acetaminophen (Percocet), oxycodone with aspirin (Percodan), oxycodone with ibuprofen (Combunox), oxymorphone (Opana, Opana ER), pentazocine (Talwin,), tapentadol (Nucynta, Nucynta ER) and tramadol and tramadol with acetaminophen (Ultram, Ultracet). Mixed opioid agonist/antagonists include: pentazocine/naloxone (Talwin NX), butorphanol and nalbuphine (Nubain).

Be aware that narcotics do not ease nerve pain.

If you have inflammatory (joint) pain or neuropathic (nerve) pain in addition to nociceptive (generalized pain) you may need an anti-inflammatory or a neuropathic medication as well.

In general, your medications may not work for the following reasons:

1. Most drugs are manufactured for a specific ailment. If your diagnosis is wrong, and if you were prescribed a specific drug for a disease, you will not receive any relief.

2. Your prescribed drug may be adversely affected by your hormones.

3. Other drugs that you are taking may interfere with your medicine. Drug-drug interactions occur when two or more drugs react with each other. Drug-food/beverage interactions result from drugs reacting with foods or beverages. Drug-condition interactions may occur when an existing medical condition makes certain drugs potentially harmful.

4. Your drug won't work if it is not absorbed by your stomach or small intestine due to excess acid in your gut.

5. Many drugs will not work unless the drug is converted into a new medication in your liver. You may have a genetic mutation which prevents this conversion.

6. Your dose of medication may not be sufficient.

7. Your medicine may not be potent enough.

8. Most drugs need to be absorbed from your stomach or small intestine to enter your blood stream. Abdominal surgery may not leave a way for a drug to get into your blood stream.

9. Your liver may filter a large portion of the drug before it gets to the proper receptor.

10. Your kidneys may excrete your drug too quickly before it has time to give you relief.

11. Some foods that you eat may interact with your medication causing your medication not to work.

12. Smoking may inhibit the effects of some medications.

13. Many medications are divided into subclasses. A change from one subclass to another subclass may be effective for your condition.

14. Other factors can affect how quickly a drug is absorbed. For example, most absorption of oral drugs occurs in the small intestine. If a patient has had large sections of the small intestine surgically removed, drug absorption decreases. If your body does not absorb enough drug, it may not work.

15. Pain and stress can also decrease the amount of drug absorbed by your body.

16. Drug tolerance occurs when a patient develops a decreased response to a drug over time. You then require a larger dose of medication to produce the same response.

17. Some generic drugs may not work as well as the brand name drugs.

18. Your gender may affect how your drug works.

19. Medications may be given by mouth, by patch, by suppository, by injection or by nasal spray. If one form of drug is ineffective another form may work.

20. Some drugs compete for the same receptor (e.g. Narcan and Morphine where Narcan pushes the Morphine off the mu receptor which stops the effects of the Morphine).

21. You must read all the instructions and warnings that come with your medication for your drug to work effectively.

Your opioid drug may not work because of the following drugs taken with your pain pill: amitriptyline, diazepam, phenytoin, protease inhibitors, and rifampin. Since a number of different compounds, (e.g., certain antihistamines, some steroids, and anti-psychotics have phencyclidine) none of which are opioid in structure but can affect receptor binding affinity for these sites. You need to be aware that smoking tobacco can also decrease the potency of hydrocodone. Long-term use of opioids can weaken your immune system and affect sex hormones that disrupt women's menstrual cycles, cause men to have difficulty achieving an erection, and reduce sexual desire in both sexes. But clinical trials suggest that short-acting versions work just as well, even for chronic pain. There is no evidence that long-acting drugs are less addictive. Moreover, long-acting versions are more likely to cause fatal overdoses, even at recommended doses.

## 18. Local Anesthetics

Sometimes your dentist needs to numb a part of your mouth. He or she injects medicine into your gum or inner cheek. This medicine is called local anesthesia. There are two kinds of numbing injections. A block injection numbs an entire region of your mouth, such as one side of your lower jaw. An infiltration injection numbs a smaller area. This is the area near where the injection was given.

Regional anesthesia is a targeted type of anesthesia. It involves injecting numbing medicine around nerves that provide sensation to specific regions or parts of your body (e.g., arm, leg, foot) for surgical procedures. Anesthesiologists can perform these procedures before surgery to prevent pain, or they can provide regional anesthesia to relieve pain after surgery. The types of regional anesthesia procedures include spinal, epidural or peripheral nerve block.

Lidocaine is the most common local anesthetic that dentists use. There are many others. Many people think of Novocain as the classic numbing drug. But Novocain actually is not used anymore. Other drugs last longer and work better than Novocain. These drugs also are less likely to cause allergic reactions.

Local anesthetics are being increasingly applied in different surgeries. Lower side effects of spinal anesthesia, regional anesthesia, and field block, in comparison to general anesthesia are the main reasons why physicians prefer to conduct surgeries under local anesthesia, especially in outpatient and day-care surgeries. Local anesthesia uses medicine to block sensations of pain from a specific area of the body. Local anesthetics are usually given by injection into the body area that needs to be anesthetized. Local anesthesia can also be applied directly to the skin or mucous membranes as a liquid or gel. This is called topical anesthesia.

Pain is described as an unpleasant sensory and emotional experience associated with actual or potential tissue damage or described in terms of such damage. Local anesthetics are numbing medicines, which can decrease your pain if you have dental work or minor surgery. The main working principle of local anesthetics is to inhibit the electric flow on nerve cell membranes to stabilize membrane potential and block painful stimulus conduction so that you will feel no pain.

Local anesthetics produce anesthesia by inhibiting excitation of nerve endings or by blocking conduction in peripheral nerves. This is achieved by anesthetics reversibly binding to and inactivating sodium channels. Sodium influx through these channels is necessary for the depolarization of nerve cell membranes and subsequent propagation of impulses along the course of the nerve. When a nerve loses depolarization and capacity to propagate an impulse, the individual loses sensation in the area supplied by the nerve.

Local anesthetics can be defined as compounds capable of reversibly suspending the ability of the nerve tissue to conduct painful stimuli. Local anesthetics differ from one another with respect how quick each drug works, and how long it lasts. When an agent and a technique are chosen for a procedure, it is important for the clinician to understand the onset, depth, and duration of anesthesia in relation to the operative procedure to be performed.

Cocaine was first used as a local anesthetic by Carl Koller and Sigmund Freud. They noticed a numbing effect on the tongue after swallowing cocaine, and Koller, who was intent on finding a drug to anaesthetize the cornea for eye surgery, knew that Freud had relieved pain with cocaine.

Local anesthetics, therefore, can be defined as compounds capable of reversibly suspending the ability of the nerve tissue to conduct painful stimuli. Local anesthetics can be divided into two chemical groups: esters and amides. Generally, allergy or hypersensitivity to an amide local anesthetic does not cross react with ester local anesthetics. This means that if you are allergic to one class of local anesthetic, you might not be allergic to the other class. Local anesthetics are therefore, into amide and ester classes. Historically, amide anesthetics (lidocaine, bupivacaine and ester procaine, tetracaine anesthetics were both used, but esters lost their favor after reports of increased sensitization. For most routine procedures in the office, amide anesthetics are used.

Amides include bupivacaine, lidocaine, mepivicaine, prilocaine, ropivacaine and etidocaine. Esters include procaine, chloroprocaine, tetracaine, cocaine, benzocaine, novocaine and procainamide. Amino esters and amino amides differ in several respects. Amino esters are metabolized in the plasma via pseudocholinesterases, whereas amino amides are metabolized in the liver. Amino esters are unstable in solution, but amino amides are very stable in solution. Amino esters are much more likely than amino amides to cause allergic hypersensitivity reactions.

Vasoconstrictors are added to local anesthetic solutions to inhibit absorption and prolong the duration of action of the anesthetic and reduce the toxicity of the anesthetic. Adrenaline is the most commonly used vasoconstrictor.

Many options to deliver anesthesia have developed over the last several decades. Administration of topical anesthetics to control pain associated with procedures such as laceration repair may avoid the need for infiltrative local anesthesia injections and associated pain from the injections. Topical anesthesia also avoids the risk of wound margin distortion that exists with infiltrative injection administration. Many local anesthetics forms exist (e.g., gels, sprays, creams, ointments, patches) and provide the clinician with local anesthetic options for application under various circumstances.

Procaine was the first compound to be used in humans. It has a relatively short duration of action. Lidocaine is currently the most widely used local anesthetic in clinical practice throughout the world. The duration of action of lidocaine is double that of procaine. Articaine introduced to medical practice in 1974, has similar potency, toxicity, and duration of action to lidocaine. Articaine is used almost exclusively in dental practice. Bupivacaine: The toxicity of bupivacaine is ten times that of procaine and has a longer duration of action than lidocaine. Mepivacaine has the potency and toxicity properties of lidocaine. This local anesthetic agent has a mild vasoconstrictor effect, which leads to a prolonged duration of action. The newest additions to clinically available local anesthetics, namely ropivacaine and levobupivacaine, which represent anesthetics, which are less toxic, more potent, and longer acting than other local anesthetics.

There are few absolute contraindications for local injection anesthetics. Allergy to amide anesthetics such as lidocaine is rare, and when it does occur, it is usually caused by the preservative methylparaben. This preservative is in the local anesthetic to keep the medicine sterile. One way to prevent a potential allergic reaction is to use preservative-free lidocaine, which is available in single-dose vials. A history of an allergy to an ester anesthetic such as procaine is not a contraindication to the use of lidocaine, because they are chemically different, and cross-reaction is rare.

Topical anesthetics are used for various skin and mucous membrane conditions, including (but not limited to) pruritus and pain due to minor burns, skin eruptions (eg, varicella, sunburn, poison ivy, insect bites), and local analgesia on intact skin. With the exception of lidocaine-prilocaine as a eutectic mixture (EMLA), topical anesthetics are poorly absorbed through the intact skin. Because of variation in systemic absorption and toxicity, the ideal choice of topical anesthetic and particular concentration depends on the intended use. EMLA has also been applied to children to minimize discomfort prior to injections or to starting an intravenous line.

Pseudocholinesterase deficiency is an inherited blood plasma enzyme abnormality. People who have this abnormality may be sensitive to certain ester anesthetic drugs.

A decrease in tissue pH shifts the anesthetic toward the ionized form which delays the onset of action. This explains why local anesthetics are slower in onset of action and less effective in the presence of inflammation, which creates a more acidic environment with a lower pH which causes ionization of the local anesthetic. On the other hand, the addition of sodium bicarbonate to the local anesthetic is used clinically to increase the pH of local anesthetic solutions thereby enhancing onset of action. Too much alkalinization of a local anesthetic, however, can cause local anesthetic molecules to precipitate from solution. Addition of epinephrine to the local anesthetic solution may improve safety and allow administration of lower doses of local anesthetic. Epinephrine may prolong the duration of the local anesthetic.

High doses of local anesthetics produce high plasma concentrations of local anesthetics, which initially produce stimulation of your brain, which may cause seizures followed by brain depression, including unconsciousness. The brain stimulatory effect may be absent in some patients, however. Solutions that contain epinephrine may add to the brain stimulatory effect as well.

You need to know that high blood levels of local anesthetics typically depress your heart and may slow your heart rate and cause you to have arrhythmias, hypotension, cardiovascular collapse, and cardiac arrest. Local anesthetics that contain epinephrine may cause hypertension, tachycardia, and angina as well.

Why won't my medications work?

There are a number of reasons why local anesthesia may not work. The reasons are: 1. poor technique by the person administrating the local anesthetic 2. Anatomical variation as a result of unusual anatomy where the injection is being performed 3.local infection in the area to be given the anesthesia. An infection in the area to be injected decreases the effect of the local anesthetic as a low pH exists and the local anesthetic is sensitive to low ph. 4. Hypersensitivity due to fear as the hormones related to anxiety (epinephrine) can prevent local anesthetics from working properly in some patients. Anesthesia works by numbing the local nerves in the oral cavity for a temporary time to make oral procedures painless and comfortable.

A reason why you may not respond to local anesthesia may be due to anatomical distribution of your nerves. In most people, anatomic structures are found in similar locations, and general rules apply, but some people's anatomy is different and since the face is such a vascularized, and complicated anatomical area that it may not be similarly distributed in everyone. A growing body of research shows that people with red hair need larger doses of anesthesia and often are resistant to local pain blockers.

A local anesthetic is always effective if it is given in the right spot and has enough time to take effect. It works by blocking the nerve supply to the particular region being treated.

However, there is huge anatomical variation between people and some people have such an unusual anatomy that the "standard" dental block used by 99% of dentists may not work. The lack of effectiveness of local anesthetic doesn't just apply to dental work, but also to pain relief during childbirth, labor (epidurals, spinals) as well.

## 19. Neuropharmacology

Anticonvulsant drugs have been used for both the management of seizures and neuropathic (damaged nerves) pain since the 1960s. These drugs interfere with the total number of pain signals that travel to your brain. The clinical impression is that they are useful for chronic neuropathic (nerve damage) pain, especially when the pain is lancinating or burning. Pain is usually the natural consequence of tissue injury resulting in approximately forty million medical appointments per annum. In general, following most injuries, as the healing process commences, the pain and tenderness associated with your injury will resolve. Unfortunately, some individuals experience pain without an obvious injury or suffer pain that persists for months or years after their initial injury. This pain condition is neuropathic in nature and accounts for a large number of patients presenting to pain clinics with chronic pain.

Following any tissue injury (nerve, muscle, bone, etc.) your nervous system sounds an alarm to your brain to make you aware that you have been injured. Rather than your nervous system functioning properly to sound an alarm regarding tissue injury, in neuropathic pain, the peripheral or central nervous systems are malfunctioning and become the cause of the pain. In other words, after your nerve has healed it may still transmit pain signals. An example is a car alarm. The alarm will sound if your vehicle is being tampered with. This is normal. Now imagine that your alarm sounds when no one is near your car. Somehow there is a short circuit. The same occurs within your nervous system.

Neuropathic pain is a complex, pain state that usually is accompanied by nerve injury. With neuropathic pain, the nerve fibers themselves may be damaged, dysfunctional or injured. These damaged nerve fibers send incorrect signals to other pain centers. The impact of nerve injury includes a change in nerve function both at the site of injury and areas around the injury. Symptoms may include: shooting and burning pain and tingling and numbness.

In order to understand the effects of anti-seizure drugs, you need to be aware that these drugs can block the ion (calcium and sodium) channels that are present throughout your nervous system. Ion channels are pore-forming proteins that help to establish and control a small electrical gradient between the inside and outside of your nerve cells. When ions flow in and out of your neuron, this electric gradient ceases and pain signals subsequently cease to be transmitted to your brain. Calcium and sodium channels are anticonvulsant drugs block the pores or channels. When these drugs drop off of these channels, you will experience pain again.

Anti-seizure drugs are frequently used in pain management. It is not known exactly how anticonvulsants work to reduce pain. They may block the flow of pain signals from the brain and spinal cord. Some anticonvulsant drugs may work better than others under certain conditions. Neuropathic pain is a form of chronic pain caused by an injury to or a disease of your peripheral or central nervous system. It does not respond well to traditional pain therapies like opioids or nonsteroidal antiinflammatory drugs.

In neuropathic pain, it has shown that a number of pathophysiological and biochemical changes take place in the nervous system as a result of an insult to a nerve. This property of the nervous system to adapt to external stimuli plays a crucial role in the onset and maintenance of pain symptoms. Carbamazepine (Tegretol), the first anticonvulsant studied in clinical trials, probably alleviates pain by decreasing conductance in sodium channels and inhibits ectopic nerve discharges. Results from clinical trials have been positive in the treatment of trigeminal neuralgia, painful diabetic neuropathy and post herpetic neuralgia with this medication.

Gabapentin (Neurontin) and pregabilin (Lyrica) have the most clearly demonstrated analgesic effects for the treatment of neuropathic pain, specifically for the treatment of painful diabetic neuropathy and postherpetic neuralgia. Based on the positive results of these studies and its favorable adverse effect profile, gabapentin or pregabilin should be considered the first choice of therapy for neuropathic pain. Evidence for the efficacy of phenytoin as an antinociceptive agent is weak to modest.

Lamotrigine (Lamictal) on the other hand, has good potential to modulate and control neuropathic pain. There is a potential for phenobarbital, clonazepam, valproic acid, topiramate, pregabalin and tiagabine to have antihyperalgesic and antinociceptive activities based on a result in animal models of neuropathic pain, but the efficacy of these drugs in the treatment of human neuropathic pain has not yet been fully determined in clinical trials. The role of anticonvulsant drugs for the treatment of neuropathic pain is evolving and has been clearly demonstrated with gabapentin and carbamazepine. Further advances to our understanding of the mechanisms underlying neuropathic pain syndromes and well-designed clinical trials should further the opportunities to establish the role of anticonvulsants in the treatment of neuropathic pain.

If you have had a direct injury to one of your nerves, you may benefit from an anticonvulsant drug. The clinical impression is that these drugs are useful for the treatment of chronic neuropathic pain, especially when the pain is lancinating or burning. There are seven drugs that are useful in neuropathic (nerve injury) pain; pregabilin (Lyrica), gabapentin (Neurontin), carbamazepine (Tegretol), valproic acid (Depakote), clonazepam (Klonopin), phenytoin (Dilantin),,zonisamide (Zonegran)) and lamotrigine (Lamictal).

Neurontin is an effective drug for the treatment of neuropathic pain, but Lyrica is becoming widely used in the management of many pain syndromes. It has fewer side effects than other anticonvulsant drugs. These drugs can be useful in the treatment of shingles, diabetic neuropathy and fibromyalgia. Reflex Sympathetic Dystrophy, diabetic neuropathy migraine headaches, sciatica, radiculitis, and pain associated with multiple sclerosis may respond to either of these drugs.

If you experience sharp shooting pain, these drugs may be helpful in decreasing your pain. If you experience side effects from either drug, other anticonvulsant medications are available. Oxcarbazepine (Trileptal), lamotrigine (Lamictal), topiramate (Topamax), and zonisamide (Zonegran) may also be effective in reducing pain caused by diabetic neuropathy and postherpetic neuralgia. Lyrica is now FDA approved in 2007 for the treatment of fibromyalgia.

Anticonvulsant drugs are effective in the treatment of chronic neuropathic pain but were not initially thought to be useful in the management of postoperative pain. However, similar to any nerve injury, surgical tissue injury is known to produce neuroplastic changes leading to spinal sensitization and the expression of nerve induced pain. Gabapentin (Neurontin) may decrease post-operative pain. The pharmacological effects of anticonvulsant drugs, which may be important for the modulation of these postoperative neural changes, include suppression of sodium channel, calcium channel and glutamate receptor activity at peripheral, spinal and supraspinal sites.

Your doctor may obtain a complete blood count and liver tests before prescribing some of these anticonvulsant drugs (e.g. Tegretol). Your doctor will give you a 4 to six-week trial of the drug. It may take the medication this length of time to exert its effects. Therefore, if you have no pain relief after several days, you should not stop the drug that was prescribed to you.

Because it takes your body time to adjust to one of these medications, your doctor must adhere to the phrase "begin low and proceed slow" which means that you should be prescribed a low dose, and this dose may be increased gradually over days to weeks. Anticonvulsant drugs are effective for the treatment of chronic pain but may also be useful for pain management following surgery.

Similar to any nerve injury, surgical tissue injury is known to produce changes leading to spinal cord sensitization, which can cause you to have pain after surgery. Gabapentin has been shown to decrease post-surgery pain. Pregabilin is effective in the treatment of diabetic neuropathy and shingles. Pregabilin binds to calcium channels of nerves, which results in a reduction of your pain. Some insurance plans do not pay for Lyrica because it is new and relatively expensive. However, it has been shown to be more cost-effective than gabapentin. This drug can cause dizziness, blurred vision, drowsiness, weight gain and swelling of your legs. This medication may decrease your platelet count as well.

Some anticonvulsant medicines can cause a decrease in your platelets, which can interfere with your ability to form a blood clot. If your platelets are too low, you will bruise easily. Gabapentin is effective in the management of oral phantom pain following a tooth extraction. Gabapentin binds to nerve calcium channels. The drug is useful in most nerve injury pain disorders. An average dose is 300 mg taken three times a day.

Tegretol is a drug that is chemically related to amitriptyline. It prevents repetitive discharges of your nerves. This medication works on sodium channels in your painful nerves. Inhibition of these sodium channels can decrease your pain sensations. An average dose is 200 mg every day. Side effects include dizziness, drowsiness, blurred vision and nausea. This medication can cause various forms of anemia and liver damage. As a result, your doctor will obtain a blood count and liver tests.

Tegretol has been shown to be effective in the treatment of trigeminal neuralgia (facial pain). Depakote is given at a dose of 250 mg twice a day. This medication can cause you to have liver failure. Your doctor will monitor your liver function closely. This medicine is used when the other anti convulsant medications have been tried but failed to provide pain relief. Side effects of this drug include nausea, vomiting loss of appetite and diarrhea. Tremors and sedation may also be associated with this medication.

Klonopin may be useful for the treatment of pain associated with the burning mouth syndrome. Klonopin is useful also for the treatment of lancinating pain associated with the phantom limb syndrome. The drug may also be useful for migraine headache prophylaxis and for the treatment of trigeminal neuralgia (facial pain). The usual dose is one mg per day. Side effects include mood disturbances and delirium. Lethargy and sedation may also be seen. This drug has a significant sedative effect. It should be initially only taken at bedtime.

Dilantin alters sodium, calcium and potassium channels in your nerves. An average dose is 300 mg three times a day. The number of side effects associated with this drug is significant. Liver damage can occur, and the drug can decrease your folic acid level in your bloodstream. A decrease in your folic acid blood level may actually cause your nerves in your arms and legs to have burning sensations.

Zonegran's mechanisms of action suggest that it could be effective in controlling neuropathic pain symptoms. It also decreases sodium channel activity on the sodium channels of your nerves. Side effects can include a decrease in your blood sodium levels, kidney stones, visual difficulties and secondary angle-closure glaucoma. A typical dose of this medication is 300 mg per day. Side effects related to this drug include agitation, anxiety, ataxia, confusion, depression, difficulty concentrating, headache, difficulty sleeping, memory problems, stomach pain as well as liver pathology. This medication may also cause weight loss. A dry mouth and flu-like syndrome may also be associated with this drug.

Lamictal also exerts its effects on sodium channels. This drug decreases the release of some pain-causing chemical from the ends of your nerves. The reason why you develop chronic pain after having acute nerve injury pain remains unclear. However, it is believed that Lamictal in addition to some of the other drugs mentioned may prevent this transformation. A typical dose will be 200 mg twice a day after starting at a low dose and going to 200 mg slowly. Adverse effects related to this drug include headaches, dizziness, blurred vision and nausea and vomiting. This medication may be of benefit in the treatment of pain associated with Reflex Sympathetic Dystrophy.

Why won't my medication work?

In general, your medications may not work for the following reasons:

1. Most drugs are manufactured for a specific ailment. If your diagnosis is wrong, and if you were prescribed a specific drug for a disease, you will not receive any relief.

2. Your prescribed drug may be adversely affected by your hormones.

3. Other drugs that you are taking may interfere with your medicine. Drug-drug interactions occur when two or more drugs react with each other. Drug-food/beverage interactions result from drugs reacting with foods or beverages. Drug-condition interactions may occur when an existing medical condition makes certain drugs potentially harmful.

4. Your drug won't work if it is not absorbed by your stomach or small intestine due to excess acid in your gut.

5. Many drugs will not work unless the drug is converted into a new medication in your liver. You may have a genetic mutation which prevents this conversion.

6. Your dose of medication may not be sufficient.

7. Your medicine may not be potent enough.

8. Most drugs need to be absorbed from your stomach or small intestine to enter your blood stream. Abdominal surgery may not leave a way for a drug to get into your blood stream.

9. Your liver may filter a large portion of the drug before it gets to the proper receptor.

10. Your kidneys may excrete your drug too quickly before it has time to give you relief.

11. Some foods that you eat may interact with your medication causing your medication not to work.

12. Smoking may inhibit the effects of some medications.

13. Many medications are divided into subclasses. A change from one subclass to another

subclass may be effective for your condition.

14. Other factors can affect how quickly a drug is absorbed. For example, most absorption of oral drugs occurs in the small intestine. If a patient has had large sections of the small intestine surgically removed, drug absorption decreases. If your body does not absorb enough drug, it may not work.

15. Pain and stress can also decrease the amount of drug absorbed by your body.

16. Drug tolerance occurs when a patient develops a decreased response to a drug over time. You then require a larger dose of medication to produce the same response.

17. Some generic drugs may not work as well as the brand name drugs.

18. Your gender may affect how your drug works.

19. Medications may be given by mouth, by patch, by suppository, by injection or by nasal spray. If one form of drug is ineffective another form may work.

20. Some drugs compete for the same receptor (e.g. Narcan and Morphine where Narcan pushes the Morphine off the mu receptor which stops the effects of the Morphine).

21. You must read all the instructions and warnings that come with your medication for your drug to work effectively.

Anticonvulsants, or anti-seizure medications, work as adjuvant analgesics. In other words, they can treat some types of chronic pain even though they are not designed for that purpose. While the main use of anti-seizure medication is preventing seizures, anticonvulsants do appear to be effective at treating certain kinds of chronic pain. These drugs may help decrease neuropathic pain, such as peripheral neuropathy, and chronic headaches such as migraines. Only a few anti-seizure medications are FDA approved for chronic pain treatment, including carbamazepine (for trigeminal neuralgia) and gabapentin and pregabilin (for postherpic neuralgia, or shingles pain).

Nerve damage (neuropathy) can be caused by many conditions, including: diabetes, high blood sugar levels which can damage nerves throughout your body. Anyone who has had chickenpox is at risk of shingles, a rash of blisters that can be painful or itchy. A condition called postherpetic neuralgia occurs if shingles pain persists after the rash disappears. Chemotherapy drugs can damage nerves, causing pain and numbness that generally begin in the tips of your toes and fingers. A herniated disk may cause nerve damage if a herniated disk in your spine squeezes a nerve passing through your vertebrae. Fibromyalgia is a chronic condition that causes pain and tenderness throughout the nerves your body.

You may not have epilepsy. You may be having events that look like seizures but are not. You may be having seizures, but something other than epilepsy is causing them. Taking antiepileptic drugs when you do not have epilepsy may not stop you from having seizures. If you do have epilepsy, the diagnosis of your seizure type may still be wrong. Seizures are hard to describe and hard to classify. Mistakes in identifying the types of seizures you have can lead to choosing the wrong drug. A drug that prevents one type of seizure may not work for another type or may even make seizures happen more often.

Some people have forms of epilepsy that simply will not respond to drug therapy. Some of these people may be candidates for epilepsy surgery. Many medicines for epilepsy can interact with other medicines you may be taking.

## 20. Psychopharmacology

Psychopharmacology is the scientific study of the effects drugs have on mood, sensation, thinking, and behavior. Psychopharmacology focuses primarily on the chemical interactions within the brain. Psychoactive drugs interact with particular target sites or receptors found in the brain to induce widespread changes in physiological or psychological functions. The use of drugs to alleviate the symptoms of mental disorders makes psychoactive agents among the most widely prescribed pharmaceuticals today.

A psychoactive drug or psychotropic substance is a chemical substance that acts primarily upon the central nervous system where it alters brain function, resulting in temporary changes in perception, mood, consciousness and behavior. In psychiatry, there are many symptoms that overlap, so the same symptom can represent more than one disorder, making diagnosis tricky and increasing the likelihood of the wrong kind of medication being prescribed. Additionally, if there are multiple diagnoses occurring together.

There are six major classes of psychiatric medications: antidepressants treat clinical depression, dysthymia, anxiety, eating disorders and borderline personality disorders, stimulants, which are used to treat disorders such as attention deficit disorder and narcolepsy and to suppress the appetite, antipsychotics, which are used to treat psychotic symptoms, such as those associated with schizophrenia or severe mania, mood stabilizers, which are used to treat bipolar disorder and schizoaffective disorder, anxiolytics, which are used to treat anxiety disorders and depressants, which are used as hypnotics, sedatives, and anesthetics, depending upon dosage.

Exposure to psychoactive drugs can cause changes to the brain that counteract or augment some of their effects; these changes may be beneficial or harmful. However, there is a significant amount of evidence that relapse rate of mental disorders negatively corresponds with length of properly followed treatment regimens (that is, relapse rate substantially declines over time), and to a much greater degree than placebo.

Psychotropic drugs operate by temporarily affecting a person's neurochemistry, which in turn causes changes in a person's mood, cognition, perception and behavior. There are many ways in which psychotropic drugs can affect the brain. Each drug has a specific action on one or more neurotransmitter or neuroreceptor in your brain.

Drugs that increase activity, in neurotransmitter systems are called agonists. They act by increasing the synthesis of one or more neurotransmitters, by reducing its reuptake from the synapses, or by mimicking the action by binding directly to the postsynaptic receptor. Drugs that reduce neurotransmitter activity are called antagonists, and operate by interfering with synthesis or blocking postsynaptic receptors so that neurotransmitters cannot bind to them.

Exposure to a psychoactive substance can cause changes in the structure and functioning of neurons, as the nervous system tries to reestablish the homeostasis disrupted by the presence of the drug. Exposure to antagonists for a particular neurotransmitter can increase the number of receptors for that neurotransmitter or the receptors themselves may become more responsive to neurotransmitters, which are called receptor sensitization.

On the other hand, overstimulation of receptors for a particular neurotransmitter may cause a decrease in both number and sensitivity of these receptors, a process called desensitization or tolerance. Sensitization and desensitization are more likely to occur with long-term exposure, although they may occur after only a single exposure. These processes are thought to play a role in drug dependence and addiction.

Physical dependence on antidepressants or anxiolytics may result in worse depression or anxiety, respectively, as withdrawal symptoms. Unfortunately, because clinical depression is often referred to simply as depression, antidepressants are often requested by and prescribed for patients who are depressed, but not clinically depressed. Psychopharmacology is the scientific study of the effects drugs have on mood, sensation, thinking, and behavior.

In psychiatry, there is a lot of symptom overlap, so the same symptom can represent more than one disorder, making diagnosis tricky and increases the likelihood of the wrong kind of medication being prescribed. If there are multiple diagnoses occurring together sometimes a medication helps one condition but makes another one worse. Medications that are commonly used in primary care or urgent care settings, such as sedatives, sleep agents and anti-depressants, may sometimes unmask a mental disorder in a vulnerable individual. These medications can occasionally have a paradoxical reaction, meaning that instead of having a calming effect, they cause disinhibition, agitation, or even psychosis.

In addition, several psychoactive substances are currently employed to treat various addictions. These include acamprosate or naltrexone in the treatment of alcoholism, or methadone or buprenorphine maintenance therapy in the case of opioid addiction.

Exposure to psychoactive drugs can cause changes to the brain that counteract or augment some of their effects; these changes may be beneficial or harmful. However, there is a significant amount of evidence that relapse rate of mental disorders negatively corresponds with length of properly followed treatment regimens and to a much greater degree than placebo.

Psychoactive drugs operate by temporarily affecting a person's neurochemistry, which in turn causes changes in a person's mood, cognition, perception and behavior. There are many ways in which psychoactive drugs can affect the brain. Each drug has a specific action on one or more neurotransmitter neuroreceptor in the brain.

As previously stated, drugs that increase activity in neurotransmitter systems are called agonists. They act by increasing the synthesis of one or more neurotransmitters, by reducing its reuptake from the synapses, or by mimicking the action by binding directly to the postsynaptic receptor. Drugs that reduce neurotransmitter activity are called antagonists, and operate by interfering with synthesis or blocking postsynaptic receptors so that neurotransmitters cannot bind to them.

Exposure to a psychoactive substance can cause changes in the structure and functioning of neurons, as the nervous system tries to re-establish the homeostasis disrupted by the presence of the drug. Exposure to antagonists for a particular neurotransmitter can increase the number of receptors for that neurotransmitter or the receptors themselves may become more responsive to neurotransmitters, which are called sensitization.

On the other hand, overstimulation of receptors for a particular neurotransmitter may cause a decrease in both number and sensitivity of these receptors, a process called desensitization or tolerance. Sensitization and desensitization are more likely to occur with long-term drug exposure, although they may occur after only a single exposure. These processes are thought to play a role in drug dependence and addiction.

Physical dependence on antidepressants or anxiolytics may result in worse depression or anxiety, respectively, as withdrawal symptoms. Unfortunately, because clinical depression is often referred to simply as depression, antidepressants are often requested by and prescribed for patients who are depressed, but not clinically depressed.

You now live in a culture where advertisements for drugs fill prime time slots on television and the pharmaceutical industry grabs every opportunity it can to influence the prescribing habits of doctors. For example, (Abilify) aripiprazole is used to treat the symptoms of schizophrenia in adults and teenagers 13 years of age and older. Abilify is advertised on television for the treatment of depression refractive to other antidepressant medications. It is also used alone or with other medications to treat symptoms of mania and depression that happen together in adults. Aripiprazole is also used as an antidepressant to treat depression when symptoms cannot be controlled by an antidepressant alone. Some of the side effects of Abilify include headache, nervousness, drowsiness, dizziness, heartburn, constipation, diarrhea, stomach pain, weight gain, increased appetite, increased salivation and pain, in the arms, legs or joints. Other side effects of Abilify include seizures, irregular heartbeat, chest pain, vision changes, unusual and uncontrollable movements, high fever, muscle stiffness, confusion, sweating and severe allergic reactions. The television adds quickly lists the side effects rapidly and in small print at the bottom of your television screen. Because of the complexity of psychoactive drugs as well as potential side effects, it is recommended that these drugs be prescribed by a psychiatrist.

Antianxiety drugs, also called anxiolytics, include some of the most commonly prescribed drugs in the United States. They are used primarily to treat anxiety disorders. The three main types of antianxiety drugs are benzodiazepines, barbiturates, and buspirone. Buspirone has a high affinity for serotonin receptors. Buspirone is used to treat generalized anxiety states.

Antidepressant and mood stabilizer drugs are used to treat disturbances in mood, characterized by depression or elation. Bipolar disorders are characterized by alternating periods of manic behavior and clinical depression and are treated with lithium and anticonvulsant drugs.

Selective serotonin reuptake inhibitors were developed to treat depression with fewer adverse reactions and are called SSRIs. SSRIs may also be useful in treating panic disorders, eating disorders, personality disorders, impulse control disorders, and anxiety disorders. SSRIs include citalopram, duloxetine, escitalopram, fluoxetine, fluvoxamine, paroxetine, sertraline, and venlafaxine.

Tricyclic antidepressants (TCA's) are also used to treat depression. They include: imipramine, nortriptyline, protriptyline, trimipramine, citalopram, duloxetine, escitalopram, fluoxetine, fluvoxamine, paroxetine, sertraline, and venlafaxine.

Lithium carbonate and lithium citrate are used to prevent or treat mania. Lithium's exact mechanism of action is unknown. Lithium is used primarily to treat acute episodes of mania and to prevent relapses of bipolar disorders.

Stimulants are used to treat attention deficit hyperactivity disorders. Examples are dextroamphetamine, lisdexamfetamine, methylphenidate, mixed amphetamine salts and modafinil. These drugs are helpful in improving attention, performance, and decreasing impulsivity and hyperactivity. Stimulants are highly abused substances, and close monitoring is required.

Be aware of drug-drug interactions. Barbiturates increase the metabolism of TCAs and decrease their blood levels. Therefore, your medication will not work as well with a decreased

TCA level. Cimetidine impairs metabolism of TCAs by the liver, increasing the risk of toxicity. An increased intake of sodium may reduce the therapeutic effects of lithium.

If you've been treated for depression but your symptoms haven't improved, you may have treatment-resistant depression. Taking an antidepressant or going to psychological counseling eases depression symptoms for most people. But with treatment-resistant depression, standard treatments aren't enough. They may not help much at all, or your symptoms may improve, only to keep coming back.

A psychiatrist will review your medical history and may inquire about life situations that might be contributing to your depression. Review all of the medications you're taking, including nonprescription drugs and herbal supplements. Make sure that you're taking your medications as prescribed and following other treatment steps. Consider a diagnosis of another mental health condition, such as bipolar disorder, which can cause or worsen depression and may require different treatment; dysthymia, a mild but long-term form of depression; or a personality disorder that contributes to the depression not getting better. Consider physical health conditions that can sometimes cause or worsen depression, such as thyroid disorders or heart problems. Give your current medications more time. Antidepressants and other medications for depression typically take four to eight weeks to become fully effective and for side effects to ease up. Increase your dose. Because people respond to medications differently, you may benefit from a higher dose of medication than is usually prescribed. Switch antidepressants. For a number of people, the first antidepressant tried isn't effective. Add another type of antidepressant. These chemicals are neurotransmitters that include dopamine, serotonin and norepinephrine. Add a medication generally used for another condition. This approach may include antipsychotics, mood stabilizers, anti-anxiety medications, thyroid hormone, beta blockers, stimulants or other drugs. Consider the cytochrome P450 genotyping test. This test checks for specific genes that indicate how well your body can process a medication. Because of inherited traits that cause variations in certain P450 enzymes, medications may affect each person differently. Psychological counseling is an important treatment as well.

What can I do if my anxiety medications are not working?

Anxiety medications do not cure anxiety. They dull the senses of in an attempt to mask the symptoms of the underlying problem. Most people find their anxiety medications not working and they continue to feel stressed and panicky to some degree. If you believe the anxiety medications you are taking are not working, or are actually making your situation worse, it is important that you first contact your doctor before taking any action or discontinuing using the medication. It is well-known that many anti-anxiety medications can have withdrawal symptoms if the user attempts to abruptly stop the medication.

If the anxiety medications are not working, there are plenty of alternative anxiety remedies you can use to restore balance back into your life by dealing with the cause of the anxiety issues It is also important to consider your diet when dealing with an anxiety problem. Reducing caffeine intake is critical for people who are prone to anxiety. Nicotine should also be avoided, as it is a stimulant and can aggravate anxiety symptoms. The simple act of reducing your daily intake of caffeine and nicotine can make a dramatic difference in your overall level of stress. Another aspect of your diet that can contribute to anxiety is food allergies. Undiagnosed food allergies can often cause mood instability and emotional problems such as anxiety and panic attacks. One of the most chronically undiagnosed food allergies is dairy products, including milk. It is possible for an individual to decrease their anxiety by eliminating dairy products from their diet. Many anti-anxiety medications are often addictive, which is why it is so important to learn how to cope with the anxiety rather than depending on medications.

Why won't my medication work?

In general, your medications may not work for the following reasons:

1. Most drugs are manufactured for a specific ailment. If your diagnosis is wrong, and if you were prescribed a specific drug for a disease, you will not receive any relief.

2. Your prescribed drug may be adversely affected by your hormones.

3. Other drugs that you are taking may interfere with your medicine. Drug-drug interactions occur when two or more drugs react with each other. Drug-food/beverage interactions result from drugs reacting with foods or beverages. Drug-condition interactions may occur when an existing medical condition makes certain drugs potentially harmful.

4. Your drug won't work if it is not absorbed by your stomach or small intestine due to excess acid in your gut.

5. Many drugs will not work unless the drug is converted into a new medication in your liver. You may have a genetic mutation which prevents this conversion.

6. Your dose of medication may not be sufficient.

7. Your medicine may not be potent enough.

8. Most drugs need to be absorbed from your stomach or small intestine to enter your blood stream. Abdominal surgery may not leave a way for a drug to get into your blood stream.

9. Your liver may filter a large portion of the drug before it gets to the proper receptor.

10. Your kidneys may excrete your drug too quickly before it has time to give you relief.

11. Some foods that you eat may interact with your medication causing your medication not to work.

12. Smoking may inhibit the effects of some medications.

13. Many medications are divided into subclasses. A change from one subclass to another subclass may be effective for your condition.

14. Other factors can affect how quickly a drug is absorbed. For example, most absorption of oral drugs occurs in the small intestine. If a patient has had large sections of the small intestine surgically removed, drug absorption decreases. If your body does not absorb enough of a drug, it may not work.

15. Pain and stress can also decrease the amount of drug absorbed by your body.

16. Drug tolerance occurs when a patient develops a decreased response to a drug over time. You then require a larger dose of medication to produce the same response.

17. Some generic drugs may not work as well as the brand name drugs.

18. Your gender may affect how your drug works.

19. Medications may be given by mouth, by patch, by suppository, by injection or by nasal spray. If one form of drug is ineffective another form may work.

20. Some drugs compete for the same receptor (e.g. Narcan and Morphine where Narcan pushes the Morphine off the mu receptor which stops the effects of the Morphine).

21. You must read all the instructions and warnings that come with your medication for your drug to work effectively.

## 21. Hypertensive Drugs

High blood pressure or hypertension is a chronic medical condition in which your blood pressure is persistently elevated. Blood pressure is the measure of the force of blood pushing against your blood vessel walls. The heart pumps blood into the arteries which carry your blood throughout your body. High blood pressure is bad because it makes the heart work harder to pump blood out to the body and contributes to hardening of the arteries, or atherosclerosis, to stroke, kidney disease, and to the development of heart failure.

Hypertension means your systolic blood pressure (top number) is consistently over 140 of your blood pressure measurement, which represents the pressure generated when your heart beats. A diastolic (bottom number) blood pressure over 90 represents the pressure in your arteries when your heart is at rest. The exact causes of high blood pressure are not known, but several factors and conditions may play a role in its development.

Doctors usually initially prescribe a single, low-dose medicine first to treat your hypertension. If your blood pressure is not controlled, your doctor may change the dosage of your medication or try a different medicine or combination of medicines. It is common to try several medicines before blood pressure is successfully controlled. Many people need more than one hypertensive medicine.

Hypertension can be caused by smoking, obesity, lack of exercise, too much salt or alcohol, stress, older age, family history of high blood pressure, kidney disease, adrenal and thyroid disorder or sleep apnea. Illegal drugs, such as cocaine and amphetamine can cause hypertension. Certain medications, such as birth control pills, cold remedies, decongestants, over-the-counter pain relievers and some prescription drugs can cause high blood pressure.

In as many as 95% of reported high blood pressure cases in the U.S., the underlying cause cannot be determined. This type of high blood pressure is called essential hypertension. When a direct cause for high blood pressure can be identified, the condition is described as secondary hypertension.

High blood pressure has many risk factors, including: Age, gender and race. The risk of high blood pressure increases as you age. Through early middle age, or about age 45, high blood pressure is more common in men. Women are more likely to develop high blood pressure after age 65. High blood pressure is common among blacks.

First line medications for hypertension include thiazide-diuretics, calcium channel blockers, angiotensin converting enzyme inhibitors and angiotensin receptor blockers. These drugs may be used alone or in combination. The majority of people require more than one medication to control their hypertension. There is a wide range of blood pressure medications available. These are grouped under four main types of medications:

Angiotensin-converting enzyme (ACE) inhibitors help relax blood vessels. ACE inhibitors prevent an enzyme in your body from producing angiotensin II, a substance in your body that affects your cardiovascular system by narrowing your blood vessels and releasing hormones that can raise your blood pressure. Examples of ACE inhibitors include: benazepril, captopril, enalapril, fosinopril, lisinopril, moexipril, perindopril, quinapril, Ramipril and trandolapril.

Angiotensin II receptor blockers (ARBs) have the same effects as ACE inhibitors, another type of blood pressure drug, but work by a different mechanism. These drugs block the effect of angiotensin II, a chemical that narrows blood vessels. By doing so, they help widen blood vessels to allow blood to flow more easily, which lowers blood pressure. ARBs are generally prescribed for people who cannot tolerate ACE inhibitors.

Calcium channel blockers are drugs used to lower blood pressure as well. They work by slowing the movement of calcium into the cells of the heart and blood vessel walls, which makes it easier for the heart to pump and widens blood vessels.

As a result, the heart doesn't have to work as hard, and blood pressure lowers. Calcium channel blockers include amlodipine, diltiazem, felodipine, isradipine, nicardipine, nifedipine, nisoldipine and verapamil.

Thiazide diuretics are sometimes called water pills which help rid your body of sodium) and water. They work by making your kidneys put more sodium into your urine. The sodium, in turn, takes water with it from your blood. That decreases the amount of fluid flowing through your blood vessels, which reduces pressure on the walls of your arteries.

Other medications used include: beta blockers. These work by blocking certain nerve and hormonal signals to the heart and blood vessels which lowers your blood pressure. Frequently prescribed beta blockers include metoprolol, nadolol and atenolol.

Renin inhibitors may also be prescribed to lower your blood pressure. Renin is an enzyme produced by your kidneys that increases your blood pressure. Aliskiren slows down the production of renin, reducing its ability to begin this process. Due to a risk of serious complications, including stroke, you shouldn't take aliskiren along with ACE inhibitors or angiotensin II receptor blockers if you have diabetes or kidney disease.

Why don't my blood pressure medications work?

# WHY WON'T MY MEDICATION WORK?

1. Most drugs are manufactured for a specific ailment. If your diagnosis is wrong, and if you were prescribed a specific drug for a disease, you will not receive any relief.

2. Your prescribed drug may be adversely affected by your hormones.

3. Other drugs that you are taking may interfere with your medicine. Drug-drug interactions occur when two or more drugs react with each other. Drug-food/beverage interactions result from drugs reacting with foods or beverages. Drug-condition interactions may occur when an existing medical condition makes certain drugs potentially harmful

4. Your drug won't work if it is not absorbed by your stomach or small intestine due to excess acid in your gut.

5. Many drugs will not work unless the drug is converted into a new medication in your liver. You may have a genetic mutation which prevents this conversion.

6. Your dose of medication may not be sufficient.

7. Your medicine may not be potent enough.

8. Most drugs need to be absorbed from your stomach or small intestine to enter your blood stream. Abdominal surgery may not leave a way for a drug to get into your blood stream.

9. Your liver may filter a large portion of the drug before it gets to the proper receptor.

10. Your kidneys may excrete your drug too quickly before it has time to give you relief.

11. Some foods that you eat may interact with your medication causing your medication not to work.

12. Smoking may inhibit the effects of some medications.

13. Many medications are divided into subclasses. A change from one subclass to another subclass may be effective for your condition.

14. Other factors can affect how quickly a drug is absorbed. For example, most absorption of oral drugs occurs in the small intestine. If a patient has had large sections of the small intestine surgically removed, drug absorption decreases. If your body does not absorb enough drug, it may not work.

15. Pain and stress can also decrease the amount of drug absorbed by your body.

16. Drug tolerance occurs when a patient develops a decreased response to a drug over time. You then require a larger dose of medication to produce the same response.

17. Some generic drugs may not work as well as the brand name drugs.

18. Your gender may affect how your drug works.

19. Medications may be given by mouth, by patch, by suppository, by injection or by nasal spray. If one form of drug is ineffective another form may work.

20. Some drugs compete for the same receptor (e.g. Narcan and Morphine where Narcan pushes the Morphine off the mu receptor which stops the effects of the Morphine).

21. You must read all the instructions and warnings that come with your medication for your drug to work effectively.

Usually, it's not just one single issue but various factors that contribute to the lack of medication efficacy. Finding the right combination of medications for uncontrolled hypertension may require some trial and error. Other drugs can interfere with blood pressure control, oral contraceptives and nasal decongestants. The low sodium DASH diet is recommended for hypertension: fruits, vegetables, whole grains and lean protein, with no more than 2.3 grams of sodium each day. To help lower your blood pressure decrease your weight, increase your physical activity only moderate alcohol consumption and quit smoking.

The etiology of resistant hypertension is almost always multifactorial; look for lifestyle aspects such as excessive sodium in the diet and moderate-to-heavy alcohol use. In addition, many commonly used medications can hamper BP control. These include selected COX-2 inhibitors (Celebrex), adrenergic drugs and stimulants, and oral contraceptives. Non-steroidal anti-inflammatory drugs may reduce the BP-lowering effects of beta-blockers, ACE-inhibitors, angiotensin II-receptor blockers (ARBs) and diuretics. Finally, consider secondary causes for resistant hypertension such as sleep apnea, renal parenchymal disease, primary or secondary aldosteronism, chronic kidney disease, renal-vascular stenosis and hypertension.

Other drugs can interfere with blood pressure control, including anti-inflammatory pain relievers. You may have other medical conditions that are affecting your blood pressure like hyperthyroidism as well.

High blood pressure is often seen in combination with other health problems. Those conditions include: heart failure, previous heart attack, and high risk of coronary artery disease, enlarged or thickened chamber of the heart, diabetes, chronic kidney disease or a previous stroke.

Medication to reduce high blood pressure may not work as well as hoped for a variety of reasons. The patient may be on the wrong drug or need additional medication. Additionally, lifestyle changes are an integral part of any hypertension treatment, and failure to do so may make blood pressure medications far less effective. Reducing salt intake is a key to decreasing high blood pressure. A hypertensive patient should ingest no more than 1,500 mg of sodium each day.

Failure to quit smoking cigarettes can make blood pressure medications ineffective. Tobacco use increases hardening of the arteries, which also worsens hypertension. Increasing potassium intake through eating fruits such as bananas and orange juice can also help reduce hypertension along with drug treatment.

## 22. Gastrointestinal Drugs

Peptic ulcers are open sores in the lining of the stomach, esophagus, or duodenum are common. According to the American College of Gastroenterology, about 20 million Americans will develop an ulcer during their life. Contrary to popular belief, ulcers are not caused by spicy food or stress. Instead, a type of bacteria called Helicobacter pylori is usually to blame. Long term use of nonsteroidal anti-inflammatory drugs (NSAIDs), such as ibuprofen, can also cause ulcers. Cigarette smoking also plays a role in the development of ulcers. Genetics, accounts for 20% to 50% of peptic ulcers. Treatments are aimed at eradicating H. pylori or restoring the balance between acid and pepsin secretions in the GI mucosa. Antacids work locally in the stomach by neutralizing gastric acid. The acid-neutralizing action of antacids reduces the total amount of acid in the GI tract, allowing peptic ulcers to heal. All antacids can interfere with the absorption of oral drugs given at the same time. Successful treatment of ulcers involves the use of two or more antibiotics in combination with other drugs such as acid suppressants.

Antiulcer drugs treat ulcers in the stomach and the upper part of the small intestine. The proton pump inhibitors block the secretion of gastric acid by the gastric parietal cells. Proton pump inhibitors disrupt chemical binding in stomach cells to reduce acid production. The extent of inhibition of acid secretion is dose related. In some cases, gastric acid secretion is completely blocked for over 24 hours on a single dose. In addition to their role in treatment of gastric ulcers, the proton pump inhibitors are used to treat syndromes of excessive acid secretion such as the Zollinger-Ellison Syndrome and gastroesophageal reflux disease (GERD). Proton pump inhibitors disrupt chemical binding in stomach cells to reduce acid production, lessening irritation and allowing peptic ulcers to heal. This class of drug includes: esomeprazole, lansoprazole, omeprazole and pantoprazole. Proton pump inhibitors may interfere with the metabolism of diazepam, phenytoin, and warfarin, causing increased half-life and elevated plasma levels of these drugs.

Other antiulcer drugs include abdominal mucosal protective agents such as sucralfate and misoprostol. Sucralfate adheres to ulcers in mucosal surfaces and aiding in healing. Sucralfate is not absorbed and has not been linked to liver injury. Sucralfate is used for the short-term treatment (up to 8 weeks) of duodenal or gastric ulcers. A secondary effect is to act as an inhibitor of the digestive enzyme pepsin . Misoprostol inhibits stomach acid secretion and aids in ulcer healing. Misoprostol is absorbed systemically, but has not been linked to liver injury.

Sucralfate does not bind to the normal stomach lining. The drug has been used for prevention of stress ulcers, the type seen in patients exposed to physical stress such as burns and surgery. It has no systemic effects. Sucralfate does not bind to the normal stomach lining. The drug has been used for prevention of stress ulcers, the type seen in patients exposed to physical stress such as burns and surgery. It has no systemic effects.

Recurrent gastric and duodenal ulcers are caused by Helicobacter pylori infections, and are treated with combination treatments that incorporate antibiotic therapy with gastric acid suppression as previously mentioned. Additionally, bismuth compounds have been used. The primary class of drugs used for gastric acid suppression is the proton pump inhibitors, omeprazole, lansoprazole, pantoprazole and rabeprazole.

Histamine H-2 receptor blockers stop the action of histamine on the gastric parietal cells, inhibiting the secretion of gastric acid. These drugs are less effective than the proton pump inhibitors, but may achieve a 75-79% reduction in acid secretion. Higher rates of acid inhibition may be achieved when the drug is administered by the intravenous route. The H-2 receptor blockers may also be used to treat heartburn syndromes. When given before surgery, the H-2 receptor blockers are useful in prevention of aspiration pneumonia. The H-2 receptor blocking agents, cimetidine, famotidine, nizatidine, and ranitidine have been used for this purpose, but are now more widely used for maintenance therapy after treatment with the proton pump inhibitors.

The proton pump inhibitors block the secretion of gastric acid by the gastric parietal cells. The extent of inhibition of acid secretion is dose related. In some cases, gastric acid secretion is completely blocked for over 24 hours on a single dose. The major, most potent and effective antiulcer medications are the selective histamine type 2 receptor blockers (H2 blockers) and the proton pump inhibitors. Both classes of antiulcer medications block the pathways of acid production or secretion, decreasing gastric acidity, improving symptoms and aiding in healing of acid-peptic diseases. These are some of the most commonly used drugs in medicine and are generally well tolerated and rarely result in serious adverse events. Nevertheless, both of these classes of agents have been linked to rare instances of acute liver injury.

Selective histamine Type 2 receptor blockers include cimetidine, famotidine, nizatidine and ranitidine. Histamine H-2 receptor blockers stop the action of histamine on the gastric parietal cells, inhibiting the secretion of gastric acid. These drugs are less effective than the proton pump inhibitors, but may achieve a 75-79% reduction in acid secretion. Higher rates of acid inhibition may be achieved when the drug is administered by the intravenous route. The H-2 receptor blockers may also be used to treat heartburn and hyper secretory syndromes. When

# WHY WON'T MY MECIDICATION WORK?

given before surgery, the H-2 receptor blockers are useful in prevention of aspiration pneumonia.

Why won't my medication work?

1. Most drugs are manufactured for a specific ailment. If your diagnosis is wrong and if you were prescribed a specific drug for a specific disease, your drug will not work.

2. Your prescribed drug may be adversely affected by your hormones.

3. Other drugs that you are taking may interfere with your medicine. Drug-drug interactions occur when two or more drugs react with each other. Drug-food/beverage interactions result from drugs reacting with foods or beverages. Drug-condition interactions may occur when an existing medical condition makes certain drugs potentially harmful. Some drugs compete for the same receptor.

4. Your drug won't work if it is not absorbed by your stomach or small intestine due to excess acid in your stomach.

5. Many drugs will not work unless the drug is converted into a new medication in your liver. You may have a genetic mutation which prevents this conversion. A genetic test can determine this.

6. Your dose of medication may not be sufficient.

7. Your medicine may not be potent enough. You may need a stronger medication.

8. Most drugs need to be absorbed from your stomach or small intestine to enter your blood stream. Previous abdominal surgery may not leave a way for a drug to get into your blood stream.

9. Your liver may filter a large portion of the drug before it gets to the proper receptor.

10. Your kidneys may excrete your drug too quickly before it has time to give you relief.

11. Some foods that you eat may interact with your medication causing your medication not to work.

12. Smoking may inhibit the effects of some medications.

13. Many medications are divided into subclasses. A change from one subclass to another subclass may be more effective for your condition.

14. Pain and stress can also decrease the amount of drugs absorbed into your body.

15. Drug tolerance occurs when a patient develops a decreased response to a drug over time. You then require a larger dose of medication to produce the same response.

16. Some generic drugs may not work as well as the brand-name drugs.

17. Your gender may affect how your drug works.

18. Medications may be given by mouth, by patch, by suppository, by injection or by nasal spray. If one form of drug is ineffective, another form may work.

19. Some drugs compete for the same receptor (e.g. Narcan and Morphine where Narcan pushes the Morphine off the mu receptor which stops the effects of the Morphine).

20. The most common reasons why your medication will not work are related to the interactions of your drug with other drugs, foods, juices, etc.

21. You must read all the instructions and warnings that come with your medication for your drug to work effectively.

With proper treatment, most ulcers heal within 6 - 8 weeks. However, they may recur, particularly if H. pylori is not treated sufficiently or if life style changes are not made. Acute duodenal ulcer treatment failure is a result of inappropriate treatment or the dose of treatment is not strong enough. Most people with H. pylori don't have any symptoms. Having H. pylori infection on the other hand, does not necessarily mean you'll have ulcers or develop stomach cancer.Long-term use of nonsteroidal anti-inflammatory drugs, such as ibuprofen, can also cause ulcers and should be discontinued or decreased if possible. Cigarette smoking also plays a role in the development of ulcers and smoking should be stopped. Alcohol use should also be stopped as well.

One-half of GERD patients don't get complete relief from the proton-pump inhibitors and most patients do not have evidence of acid erosion when doctors examine their esophagus with an endoscope. Gastroenterologists have dubbed this condition non-erosive reflux diseases, or NERD. Doctors suspect some NERD patients may be suffering from a reflux of bile, a digestive liquid produced in the liver, or from hypersensitivity to sensations in the esophagus.

Many conditions cause symptoms that mimic those of gastroesophageal reflux disease and include muscle contractions and non-acidic reflux in the esophagus. Stomach acid plays a key role in sanitizing the digestive tract and in killing off the bacteria that produce nitrosamines, a chemical compound that has been associated with an increased risk of gastric cancer.

## 23. Diabetes and Thyroid Drugs

Diabetes is the seventh leading cause of death in the United States as of 2010. Diabetes contributes to kidney disease, strokes, heart attacks, hypertension and blindness if not adequately treated. It can be a difficult disease to treat.

The first treatment for type 2 diabetes is blood sugar control is meal planning, weight loss, and exercise. The pancreas is an organ that makes insulin. Beta cells in the pancreas make insulin that gets cells in your body to use glucose for energy. With each meal, beta cells release insulin to help the body use or store the blood glucose, the body's main source of energy. In people with type 1 diabetes a condition characterized by high blood-glucose levels is caused by the body's lack of insulin. This occurs when the body's immune system attacks the insulin-producing beta cells in the pancreas and destroys them. The pancreas subsequently produces minimal or no insulin.

Type 1 diabetes develops most often in young people but can appear in adults as well. The pancreas does not produce insulin. The beta cells have been destroyed, and patients need insulin shots for their bodies to use glucose. The food you eat gets digested and broken down into a sugar your body's cells can use. This is glucose, one of the simplest forms of sugar.

Patients with type 2 diabetes make insulin, but their bodies don't respond to it. Some people with type 2 diabetes have high blood-glucose levels caused by either a lack of insulin or the body's inability to use insulin efficiently. Type 2 diabetes develops most often in middle-aged and older adults. These patients need pills or insulin shots to help their bodies use glucose.

Insulin, a pancreatic hormone, and oral antidiabetic drugs are classified as hypoglycemic drugs because they lower blood-glucose levels.

There are different types of insulin. Rapid-acting insulin is a type of insulin that starts to lower blood glucose within 5 to 10 minutes after injection and has its strongest effect 30 minutes to 3 hours after injection, depending on the type used. Aspart insulin and lispro insulin begin to work about 15 minutes after injection and peaks in 1 hour, and works for 2 to 4 hours.

Insulin isn't effective when taken orally. All insulins, however, may be given by subcutaneous injection or intravenous injection.

Regular or short-acting insulin is a type of insulin that starts to lower blood glucose within 30 minutes after injection and has its strongest effect 2 to 5 hours after injection. Regular insulin usually reaches the bloodstream within 30 minutes after injection, peaks 2 to 3 hours after injection, and is effective for 3 to 6 hours. Two types include: Humulin R and Novolin R insulin.

Intermediate-acting insulin is a type of insulin that starts to lower blood glucose within 1 to 2 hours after injection and has its maximum effect 6 to 12 hours after injection, depending on the type used. Types include NPH (Humulin N and Novolin N). Lente insulin and NPH insulin generally reach the bloodstream about 2 to 4 hours after injection, peaks 4 to 12 hours later, and is effective for about 12 to 18 hours. Types: NPH (Humulin N, Novolin N)

Long-acting insulins lower blood glucose within 4 to 6 hours after injection and have a maximum effect 10 to 18 hours after injection. Long-acting insulins reach the bloodstream several hours after injection and tend to lower glucose levels over a 24-hour period. Types include insulin Levemir) and insulin Lantus. Insulin-responsive tissues are located in the liver, adipose tissue, and muscle.

Anabolic steroids, salicylates, alcohol, and monoamine oxidase inhibitors (MAOIs) may increase the hypoglycemic effect of insulin. On the other hand, steroids, sympathomimetic drugs, thiazide diuretics, and dextrothyroxine may reduce the effects of insulin, resulting in hyperglycemia.

Your chances of lowering your blood sugar are low if you have had diabetes for more than 10 years or already take more than 20 units of insulin each day. On the other hand, your chances are good if you developed diabetes recently or have needed little or no insulin to keep your blood glucose levels near normal.

Diabetic pills sometimes stop working after a few months or years. The cause is often unknown. This doesn't mean your diabetes is worse but you may build tolerance to your medication over time. When this happens, oral combination therapy is the use of different medicines together such as oral hypoglycemic agents or an oral hypoglycemic agent and insulin to manage the blood-glucose levels with type 2 diabetes. Oral antidiabetic drugs are indicated for patients with type 2 diabetes if diet and exercise can't control blood-glucose levels. These drugs aren't effective in patients with type 1 diabetes because the patients' pancreatic beta cells aren't functioning at a minimal level. Oral antidiabetic drugs can decrease liver production and intestinal absorption of glucose and improve insulin sensitivity, delay glucose absorption, or increase insulin secretion. An antidiabetic drug may work by: stimulating the pancreas to produce and release more insulin, inhibiting the production and release of glucose from the liver, blocking the action of stomach enzymes that break down carbohydrates, improve the sensitivity of cells to insulin and inhibit the reabsorption of glucose in the kidneys.

There is no best treatment for type 2 diabetes. A patient may need to try more than one type of pill, combination of pills, or pills plus insulin.

Oral antidiabetic drugs stimulate pancreatic beta cells to release insulin. They can go to work in the liver and decrease glucose production. These drugs also increase the number of insulin receptors in the peripheral tissues and they provide more opportunities for the cells to bind sufficiently with insulin. Generally, metformin is the first medication prescribed for type 2 diabetes. If metformin and lifestyle changes aren't enough to control your blood-sugar level, other oral or injected medications can be added.

Types of diabetic pills are as follows: Precose, (acarbose) blocks enzymes that help digest sugars and slow the rise in blood sugar. It belongs to a group of drugs called alpha-glucosidase inhibitors. Dymelor (acetohexamide) lowers blood sugar by prompting the pancreas to release more insulin. Nesina (alogliptin) increases insulin levels when blood sugars are too high. Invokana (Canagliflozin) influences how much glucose leaves your body in urine, and blocks your kidney from reabsorbing glucose.

Diabinese (chlorpropamide) lowers blood sugar by prompting the pancreas to release more insulin. Welchol (colesevelam) lowers cholesterol and improves blood sugar control in adults with type 2 diabetes. Farxiga (dapagliflozin) increases how much glucose leaves the body in your urine, and inhibits your kidneys from reabsorbing glucose. Jardiance: Boosts how much glucose leaves your body in urine, and blocks your kidney from reabsorbing glucose. Amaryl (glimepiride): lowers blood sugar by prompting the pancreas to release more insulin. Glucotrol (glipizide): also lowers blood sugar by prompting the pancreas to release more insulin. DiaBeta, Glynase PresTab, Micronase (glyburide): lower blood sugar by stimulating the pancreas to release more insulin. Tradjenta (trident) increases insulin levels when blood sugars are too high, and causes the liver to decrease sugar production. Fortamet, Glucophage, Glucophage XR, Glumetza, Riomet (metformin) improve the insulin's ability to move sugar into cells. Glyset (miglitol) inhibits enzymes that break down sugars. Starlix (nateglinide) causes the pancreas to release more insulin. Actos (pioglitazone) makes fat cells more sensitive to insulin's effects. Prandin (repaglinide) causes the pancreas to release more insulin. Avandia (rosiglitazone) enables insulin be more efficient in muscle and fat. Onglyza (saxagliptin) increases insulin levels when blood sugars are elevated. Januvia (sitagliptin) increases insulin levels when blood sugars are high and decreases liver sugar production. Tolinase (tolazamide) and Orinase (tolbutamide) decrease blood sugar by stimulating the pancreas to release insulin. Several diabetes pills combine two medications of these medications into one tablet. Combinations of multiple oral antidiabetic drugs or an oral antidiabetic drug with insulin therapy may be indicated for some patients who don't respond to either therapy alone. If you've had type 2 diabetes for six to 10 years, or take over 20 units of insulin a day, your chances may be lower, but your chances of success with pills are good if you've recently developed diabetes and haven't needed insulin to keep your blood-glucose levels normal.

You may have insulin resistance if your insulin does not lower your blood sugar. Insulin resistance means that you have to use more insulin for glucose to go inside your cells, and what we think that does over time is that it may burn out the pancreas. It may make the body unable to make quite enough insulin to help the glucose go into the cells. So, insulin resistance is a resistance to the effectiveness of insulin to get glucose into the cells.

Diabetic pills can stop working. Your doctor will want to know if there have been any changes in your daily routine. Any change in your level of physical activity, a recent illness, or weight gain can cause problems with the effectiveness of your diabetes medication. A new medication that is not related to diabetes could counteract the effects of your diabetes medication.

If you've ruled out all the other potential reasons for sudden high blood sugars, it may signal that there's been a natural decline in your pancreas beta cell function. The function of the beta cells declines over time in diabetics. Patients with Type 2 diabetes will need more medication over time. Ultimately, they may require insulin to control their blood sugar. There has to be a total lifestyle change if you are diabetic. You must be diligent about your diet and exercise.

If you are not where you want to be in terms of your blood sugar and your weight, it's time to consult your doctor about what other medication options are needed. Diabetic medications can stop working. Any change in your level of physical activity, a recent illness, or even weight gain all have the potential to cause problems with the effectiveness of diabetes medication. A new medication that is not related to diabetes could also counteract the effects of your diabetes medication.

If all potential reasons for sudden high blood sugars, it may signal that there's been a natural decline in your beta cell function. The function of pancreatic beta cells decline over time in diabetic patients. The typical course in a patient with Type 2 diabetes is that they will need more medication over time. Ultimately, they may need insulin to control their blood sugar.

Remember that your medication is not meant to do it all when you are diagnosed with diabetes. You must have a total lifestyle change which means that you must be cautious about diet and exercise. You may need to ask your physician if more medications are needed. Remember that a Type 2 diabetic may need to be treated with insulin at some point in his/ her life.

Hypothyroidism calls for a lifelong regimen of thyroid replacement. No surgical techniques, alternative medicine, or conventional drugs can increase the thyroid's hormone production once it slows down. Doctors generally prescribe synthetic forms of thyroid hormone, such as levothyroxine. Thyroid drugs can be natural or synthetic hormones and may contain triiodothyronine (T3), thyroxine (T4), or both. The principal pharmacologic effect is an increased metabolic rate in body tissues. Thyroid hormones affect protein and carbohydrate metabolism and stimulate protein synthesis.

Some people also seem to need supplemental T3 in addition to T4, to feel well. While controversial, some studies have shown that patients have improvement in overall symptoms when they add T3 to their treatment. Your doctor can assess the amount of thyroid hormone needed by doing a thyroid-stimulating hormone test (TSH test) to determine your response to the thyroid medication.

If your thyroid medication does not work you may have an adrenal gland insufficiency. Unless the adrenal problem is identified and addressed, the thyroid medication is may not be effective. Your doctor can assess your adrenal function with laboratory testing. Cholestyramine and colestipol reduce the absorption of thyroid hormones, and your thyroid medications become ineffective. Carbamazepine, phenytoin, phenobarbital, and rifampin increase the metabolism of thyroid hormones, which reduces their effectiveness.

Why won't my medication work?

1. Most drugs are manufactured for a specific ailment. If your diagnosis is wrong and if you were prescribed a specific drug for a specific disease, your drug will not work.

2. Your prescribed drug may be adversely affected by your hormones.

3. Other drugs that you are taking may interfere with your medicine. Drug-drug interactions occur when two or more drugs react with each other. Drug-food/beverage interactions result from drugs reacting with foods or beverages. Drug-condition interactions may occur when an existing medical condition makes certain drugs potentially harmful. Some drugs compete for the same receptor.

4. Your drug won't work if it is not absorbed by your stomach or small intestine due to excess acid in your stomach.

5. Many drugs will not work unless the drug is converted into a new medication in your liver. You may have a genetic mutation which prevents this conversion. A genetic test can determine this.

6. Your dose of medication may not be sufficient.

7. Your medicine may not be potent enough. You may need a stronger medication.

8. Most drugs need to be absorbed from your stomach or small intestine to enter your blood stream. Previous abdominal surgery may not leave a way for a drug to get into your blood stream.

9. Your liver may filter a large portion of the drug before it gets to the proper receptor.

10. Your kidneys may excrete your drug too quickly before it has time to give you relief.

11. Some foods that you eat may interact with your medication causing your medication not to work.

12. Smoking may inhibit the effects of some medications.

13. Many medications are divided into subclasses. A change from one subclass to another subclass may be more effective for your condition.

14. Pain and stress can also decrease the amount of drugs absorbed into your body.

15. Drug tolerance occurs when a patient develops a decreased response to a drug over time. You then require a larger dose of medication to produce the same response.

16. Some generic drugs may not work as well as the brand-name drugs.

17. Your gender may affect how your drug works.

18. Medications may be given by mouth, by patch, by suppository, by injection or by nasal spray. If one form of drug is ineffective, another form may work.

19. Some drugs compete for the same receptor (e.g. Narcan and Morphine where Narcan pushes the Morphine off the mu receptor which stops the effects of the Morphine).

20. The most common reasons why your medication will not work are related to the interactions of your drug with other drugs, foods, juices, etc.

21. You must read all the instructions and warnings that come with your medication for your drug to work effectively.

## 24. Chemotherapy

Chemotherapy is the use of anticancer drugs designed to slow or stop the growth of rapidly dividing cancer cells in the body. Given alone or with other drugs, cancer drugs may effectively act against various malignant neoplasms. The goal of chemotherapy is to stop a tumor from growing and to stop cancer from recurring and spreading to other parts of the body. There are many different types of chemotherapy. If one drug doesn't work your oncologist will most likely try another drug. This is quite common either because the body becomes sensitized to a chemotherapy drug and it stops working, or because the side effects are too hard to tolerate.

These drugs fall into one of six classes: nitrogen mustards, alkyl sulfonates, nitrosoureas, triazenes, ethylenimines and alkylating-like drugs. Alkylating agents directly damage DNA to keep the cell from reproducing. These drugs work in all phases of the cell cycle and are used to treat many different cancers, including leukemia, lymphoma, Hodgkin disease, multiple myeloma, and sarcoma, as well as cancers of the lung, breast, and ovary. Antimetabolites interfere with DNA and RNA growth by substituting for the normal building blocks of RNA and DNA. These agents damage cells during the phase, when the cell's chromosomes are being copied. They are commonly used to treat leukemia, cancers of the breast, ovary, and the intestinal tract, as well as other types of cancer. Anti-tumor antibiotics are like the antibiotics used to treat infections. They work by altering the DNA inside cancer cells to keep them from growing and multiplying. Anthracyclines are anti-tumor antibiotics that interfere with enzymes involved in DNA replication. These drugs work in all phases of the cell cycle. Topoisomerase inhibitors are used to treat certain leukemias, as well as lung, ovarian, gastrointestinal, and other cancers. Mitotic inhibitors are often plant alkaloids and other compounds derived from natural products. Drugs in this category are sex hormones, or hormone-like drugs, that change the action or production of female or male hormones. They are used to slow the growth of breast, prostate, and endometrial (uterine) cancers, which normally grow in response to natural sex hormones in the body. Some drugs are given to people with cancer to help their immune systems recognize and attack cancer cells. When looking at how to best combine two or more chemo drugs, doctors must also consider potential interactions between the drugs. They have to look at interactions between chemo drugs and other medicines the person is taking, too, including vitamins and nonprescription medicines. In some patients, these interactions may make side effects worse. In others, they may interfere with how well the chemo works.

Chemotherapy was first used to treat cancer in the 1950s. It has helped many people live full lives. There are more than 100 chemotherapy drugs used today. Doctors choose certain drugs based on the kind of cancer you have and how much cancer is in your body. New therapeutic medications such as monoclonal antibodies or targeting specific proteins are further increasing the time that a patient's cancer can remain in remission. In addition, drugs such as interferons are being used to treat patients with cancer.

Chemotherapeutic drugs unfortunately do not work on all cancers. Chemotherapy has become more effective for the treatment of some cancers over the past thirty years. Chemotherapy kills cancer cells. These drugs can affect normal cells as well, but most normal cells can repair themselves. At some point, however, for many cancer patients, it becomes clear that chemotherapy has ceased to be effective. At this point, the goal of medicine becomes making the patient comfortable and pain-free. This is known as palliative care.

Problems with chemotherapy include the lack of specificity of cells affected by these medications. This means that a chemotherapeutic medication for the treatment of a certain cancer will not only affect the cancer cell but may damage other noncancerous cells as well. When chemotherapy drugs travel through the bloodstream to reach cells throughout your body, it is called systemic chemotherapy.

Alkylating drugs, given alone or with other drugs, effectively act against various malignant neoplasms. These drugs produce their antineoplastic effects by damaging deoxyribonucleic acid (DNA). They halt DNA's replication process by cross-linking its strands so that amino acids don't pair up correctly and cancer cells do not replicate. Nitrogen mustards form covalent bonds with DNA molecules in a chemical reaction known as alkylation. Alkylated DNA can't replicate properly, thereby resulting in cancer cell death. Nitrogen mustards are effective against malignant lymphoma, multiple myeloma, melanoma and cancers of the breast, ovaries, uterus, lung, brain, testes, bladder, prostate, and stomach. Alkyl sulfonate, has historically been used to treat chronic myelogenous leukemia, polycythemia vera, and other myeloproliferative disorders. It's also used for treatment of leukemia during bone marrow transplant procedures. Nitrosoureas are alkylating agents that work by halting cancer cell reproduction. Dacarbazine, a triazene, functions as an alkylating drug after being activated by the liver. Thiotepa, an ethylenimine derivative, is a multifunctional alkylating drug. Alkylating-like drugs are heavy metal complexes that contain platinum. Because their action resembles that of a bifunctional alkylating drug, they are referred to as alkylating-like drugs.

Antimetabolites differ sufficiently from DNA base pairs in how they interfere with this synthesis. Although researchers have developed many folic acid analogues, the early compound methotrexate remains the most commonly used. It inhibits DNA and RNA synthesis. This causes cancer cell death. Pyrimidine analogues are a diverse group of drugs that inhibit production of pyrimidine nucleotides necessary for DNA synthesis. Purine analogues are incorporated into DNA and RNA, interfering with nucleic acid synthesis and replication. Antibiotic antineoplastic drugs are antimicrobial products that produce tumoricidal effects by binding with DNA. Hormonal therapies and hormone modulators prove effective against hormone-dependent tumors, such as cancers of the prostate, breast, and endometrium. Aromatase inhibitors prevent androgen from being converted into estrogen in postmenopausal women, thereby blocking estrogen's ability to activate cancer cells; limiting the amount of estrogen means that less estrogen is available to reach cancer cells and make them grow. Antiestrogens bind to estrogen receptors and block estrogen action.

When chemotherapy drugs are directed to a specific area of the body, it is called regional chemotherapy. Some newer anticancer drugs are not generally cytotoxic, but rather target proteins that are abnormally expressed in cancer cells and that are essential for their growth. Chemotherapy kills cells that are in the process of splitting into two new cells. You need to be aware that cells in your normally body divide into more cells. However, cancer cells divide faster than non-cancer cells. If you have cancer, the cells keep on dividing until there is a mass of cells which become a tumor.

Some chemotherapy drugs kill dividing cancer cells by damaging the part of the cell's nucleus that makes it divide. Other chemotherapy drugs interrupt chemical processes involved in cell division. The main ways you can have chemotherapy are as follows: An injection into your bloodstream, an intravenous infusion into your bloodstream through a vein, or by tablets and or capsules.

In general, chemotherapy treatments damage cells as they divide. In the center of cell is a nucleus. The nucleus tells your cells to divide in order to make more cells. There are genes within your nucleus. Cancer cells are more prone to be destroyed by chemotherapeutic agents when compared to your normal cells. In other words, your normal cells are much less likely to be damaged by chemotherapy than your cancer cells.

Generally most of your cells in your body divide in order to form new cells. Because these tissues have dividing cells they can possibly be damaged by chemotherapy. However, your normal cells can replace or repair your healthy cells that are damaged by chemotherapy. Most side effects from chemotherapy treatments disappear once your treatment is finished.

Examples of cancers where chemotherapy works very well are choriocarcinoma, testicular cancer, Wilms' tumor, some disseminated lymphomas, multiple myeloma, polycythemia vera, some leukemia's and Hodgkin lymphoma. It is important to know that with respect to some cancers, that chemotherapy will not cure the cancer but can help in combination with other types of treatment. Chemotherapy may be used to shrink tumors before surgery or radiation.

It may be used after surgery or radiation to help kill any cancer cells that are left. For example, many people with breast or bowel cancer have chemotherapy after surgery to help lower the risk of the cancer returning. With some cancers, if a cure is unlikely, your doctor may suggest chemotherapy to: shrink the tumor, relieve symptoms and extend your life by controlling the cancer or putting it into remission.

Remission means that after treatment there is no sign of the cancer in the body. Complete remission means that the cancer can't be detected on scans, X-rays, or blood tests, etc. Partial remission means the treatment has killed some of the cells, but not all. The cancer has shrunk, but can still be seen on scans and doesn't appear to be growing. The treatment may have stopped the cancer from growing.

You may have chemotherapy before surgery. The aim is to shrink your cancer so that you need less extensive surgery or to make it easier for your surgeon to remove most or all of the cancer. Shrinking the cancer with chemotherapy may also mean that you can have radiotherapy to a smaller area of your body which causes les damage to your normal tissues.

Different chemotherapy drugs work on different types of cancer as stated at the beginning of this chapter. As a result, the chemotherapy drugs that you may need for a breast cancer tumor that has spread to your lungs might be different to the chemotherapy drug you would have been prescribed for a cancer that began in your breast.

If your chemotherapy drug comes as tablets or capsules that you swallow, you can take chemo therapy in your home. You will need to have regular visits to the hospital outpatient department for blood tests and checkups or to your oncologist's office.

If you are having continuous, low dose chemotherapy you may have an infusion pump that you can wear at home. If your chemotherapy is given into a vein, it is usually done in the hospital chemotherapy day clinic or on a day hospital oncology ward

Strong chemotherapy described as myelosuppressive therapy can lower the number of infection-fighting white blood cells called neutrophils in your body. White blood cells help protect your body against infection. Pegfilgrastim is a prescription medication that can help reduce your risk of infection during strong chemotherapy. It does this by boosting the number of certain infection fighting white blood cells called neutrophils, which strengthens your immune system.

Nitrogen mustards represent the largest group of alkylating drugs. Because they produce leukopenia (reduced number of white blood cells, the nitrogen mustards are effective in treating malignant neoplasms, such as Hodgkin's disease and leukemia. Busulfan, an alkyl sulfonate, has historically been used to treat chronic myelogenous leukemia, polycythemia vera. Nitrosoureas are alkylating agents that work by halting cancer cell reproduction.

In summary chemotherapy can be beneficial in some but not all cancers. Your oncologist will prescribe the medications that will help you the most and decide if chemo therapy is appropriate treatment for your cancer. Studies have discovered that chemotherapy appeared in many cases to successfully kill tumor cells and temporarily stop the growth and spread of cancer, but the treatment ultimately failed to prevent new tumors from forming. And the offender was cancer stem cells that persisted long after the chemotherapy, which quietly prompted the re-growth of new tumors at a later time. Traditional therapies like surgery, chemotherapy, and radiation do not destroy the small number of cells driving the cancer's growth. If the stem cells were eliminated, the cancer would be unable to grow and spread to other locations in the body.

When a cell goes through the cell cycle, it reproduces 2 new identical cells. Each of the 2 cells made from the first cell can go through this cell cycle again when new cells are needed. The cell cycle is important because many chemotherapy drugs work only on cells that are actively reproducing not cells that are in the resting stage. Some drugs specifically attack cells in a particular phase of the cell cycle. Chemotherapy drugs can't tell the difference between reproducing cells of normal tissues and cancer cells. This means normal cells are damaged along with the cancer cells, which can cause side effects.

Why won't my chemotherapy medications work?

1. Most drugs are manufactured for a specific ailment. If your diagnosis is wrong and if you were prescribed a specific drug for a specific disease, your drug will not work.

2. Your prescribed drug may be adversely affected by your hormones.

3. Other drugs that you are taking may interfere with your medicine. Drug-drug interactions occur when two or more drugs react with each other. Drug-food/beverage interactions result from drugs reacting with foods or beverages. Drug-

# WHY WON'T MY MECDICATION WORK?

condition interactions may occur when an existing medical condition makes certain drugs potentially harmful. Some drugs compete for the same receptor.

4. Your drug won't work if it is not absorbed by your stomach or small intestine due to excess acid in your stomach.

5. Many drugs will not work unless the drug is converted into a new medication in your liver. You may have a genetic mutation which prevents this conversion. A genetic test can determine this.

6. Your dose of medication may not be sufficient.

7. Your medicine may not be potent enough. You may need a stronger medication.

8. Most drugs need to be absorbed from your stomach or small intestine to enter your blood stream. Previous abdominal surgery may not leave a way for a drug to get into your blood stream.

9. Your liver may filter a large portion of the drug before it gets to the proper receptor.

10. Your kidneys may excrete your drug too quickly before it has time to give you relief.

11. Some foods that you eat may interact with your medication causing your medication not to work.

12. Smoking may inhibit the effects of some medications.

13. Many medications are divided into subclasses. A change from one subclass to another subclass may be more effective for your condition.

14. Pain and stress can also decrease the amount of drugs absorbed into your body.

15. Drug tolerance occurs when a patient develops a decreased response to a drug over time. You then require a larger dose of medication to produce the same response.

16. Some generic drugs may not work as well as the brand-name drugs.

17. Your gender may affect how your drug works.

18. Medications may be given by mouth, by patch, by suppository, by injection or by nasal spray. If one form of drug is ineffective, another form may work.

19. Some drugs compete for the same receptor (e.g. Nacan and Morphine where Narcan pushes the Morphine off the mu receptor which stops the effects of the Morphine).

20. The most common reasons why your medication will not work are related to the interactions of your drug with other drugs, foods, juices, etc.

21. You must read all the instructions and warnings that come with your medication for your drug to work effectively.

Chemotherapy has appeared in many cases to successfully kill tumor cells and temporarily stop the growth and spread of cancer, but the treatment ultimately failed to prevent new tumors from forming. Cancer stem cells that persisted long after chemotherapy eventually prompted the re-growth of new tumors. It appears that cancer tumors possess an inherent ability to produce their own stem cells, which can circulate throughout the body and eventually develop into tumors.

Calcium-containing drugs and foods, such as antacids and dairy products, reduce absorption of estramustine. Corticosteroids can reduce the effects of some nitrogen mustards medications.. Some other medicines can affect your chemotherapy and make it less effective. Acai berry, cumin, herbal tea, turmeric and long-term use of garlic which are all herbal supplements commonly believed to be beneficial to your health – may negatively impact chemotherapy treatment. Some herbs can interfere with the metabolism of the drugs, making them less effective.

Vitamins and minerals may appear to be safe but vitamin supplements may adversely affect chemotherapy efficacy. It is a good idea to let your health care provider know what supplements (including herbal remedies) you're taking. There's an increased risk of bleeding when busulfan is taken with anticoagulants or aspirin. If a patient is taking busulfan, anticoagulants or aspirin must be discussed with patient's doctor before continuing to do so.

## 25. Antibiotic and Antiviral Medications

Antibiotics are powerful medicines that fight bacterial infections. Used properly, antibiotics can save lives. They either kill bacteria or keep them from reproducing. The first breakthrough in antibiotics came with the discovery of penicillin by Alexander Fleming in 1928. Antibiotics can kill bacteria. However, for the antibiotic to work, it must be specific for the bacteria that it trying to destroy. Another antibiotic will not work. Overuse of antibiotics is however, one of the main causes of antibiotic resistance. Antibacterial antibiotics are commonly classified based on their mechanism of action, chemical structure, or spectrum of activity.

Viruses do not respond to antibiotics. In other words, anti-bacterial medications will not work on a viral infection. A viral infection may or may not cause a fever. For therapy to be effective, an adequate concentration of the antimicrobial must be delivered to the infection site. Some antibiotics are administered parenterally (not by mouth) because they aren't absorbed from the GI tract. Antimicrobial therapy should be modified, if possible, based on results of culture and sensitivity testing to agents). A bacterial illness frequently causes a fever. The main difference between viruses and bacteria is that viruses are packets of genetic material and cannot survive on their own, while bacteria are single-celled organisms that can survive on their own. Bacteria take in nutrients, expel waste, grow, and reproduce. Viruses need a host cell (a bacterium, or a plant or animal cell) in order to reproduce copies of itself and have no need to feed or grow in the typical sense. In fact, many argue that viruses are not living entities, just bits of genetic material and cellular machinery.

Perhaps the most important distinction between bacteria and viruses is that antibiotic drugs usually kill bacteria, but they aren't effective against viruses. Infections caused by bacteria include: Strep throat, tuberculosis and urinary tract infections. Inappropriate use of antibiotics has helped create strains of bacterial disease that are resistant to treatment with different types of antibiotic medications. Antibacterial drugs are drugs that inhibit the growth of bacteria and are used mainly to treat the whole body rather than a localized area of a bacterial infection. The usefulness of antimicrobial drugs is limited by pathogens that may develop resistance to a drug's action.

Diseases caused by viruses include: Chickenpox, AIDS, and common colds. The key difference between viral and bacterial infection is that bacterial infections increase neutrophils (a type of white cell in your blood stream. Antibiotics do not kill viruses and using them to treat viral infections causes antibiotic resistance. This means that if you develop a certain bacterial infection, the antibiotic will not work to kill the bacteria.

There are only a few antiviral medications available to treat very specific viruses, and they are not always effective. However, there are vaccines available to help prevent many infections. If you have a minor illness, and your health care provider tells you that it is a viral infection, the best thing to do is to treat the symptoms if you are able to and just let it run its course. Bacteria can increase eosinophil counts while viruses increase lymphocyte counts in your blood stream.

A bacterium is a cell, with its own metabolism, which can act independently of a host cell. A virus is composed of some form of nucleic acid (either DNA or RNA) with or without some form of protein shell. It has no metabolism of its own and can only be biologically active inside the cell of some other organism, and must take over its host cell's cellular machinery. A virus and a bacterium are also different in how a host is attacked.

Bacteria exist in abundance in both living hosts and in soil, water, etc. By their nature, they can be either beneficial or (harmful for the health of plants, humans, and other animals that come into contact with them. A virus is acellular has no cell structure and requires a living host to survive, and it causes illness in its host, which causes an immune response. Bacteria are alive, while scientists are not yet sure if viruses are living or nonliving.

Infections caused by harmful bacteria can almost always be cured with antibiotics. While some viruses can be vaccinated against, most, such as HIV and the viruses which cause the common cold, are incurable, even if their symptoms can be treated, meaning the living host must have a strong enough immune system to survive the infection. Vaccines prevent the spread and antiviral medications help to slow reproduction but cannot stop it completely.

Antibiotics are mainly of two types, those that kill bacteria and those that inhibit bacterial growth. Narrow spectrum antibiotics affect particular bacteria whereas large spectrum antibiotics affect a wide range of bacteria.

Viruses are the smallest and simplest life form known. They are 10 to 100 times smaller than bacteria. Antibiotics are compounds that are effective in treating infections caused by organisms such as bacteria, fungi and protozoa. Antibiotics are mostly small molecules, less than 2000 Daltons. Obtaining an accurate infectious disease diagnosis is necessary prior to prescribing an antibiotic.

Vaccines are compounds that are used to provide immunity to a particular disease. Vaccines are usually dead or inactivated organisms or compounds purified from them.

Viruses are the smallest type of infectious agents. They are effectively collections of large molecules. Viruses are tiny organisms that may lead to mild to severe illnesses in humans, animals and plants. Viruses, like bacteria are found almost everywhere; in the soil, in the air, on surfaces or in animals and plants. They are looking for a host organism to infect so that they can use the machinery in the cell to multiply and create more viruses. This may include flu or a cold to something more life threatening like HIV/AIDS. Whether viruses are truly alive is debatable, because they possess a much simpler structure and methods of multiplication than even the simplest bacteria, which are held to be the simplest type of life. Under certain conditions, however, viruses can self-replicate, or reproduce. There are huge amounts of viruses, exceeding every living organism put together. Not all viruses cause disease, although many do. Antivirals are medications that keep viruses from reproducing inside the body. Like antibiotics for bacteria, specific antivirals are used for specific viruses. Most of the antiviral drugs now available are designed to help deal with HIV, herpes viruses, the hepatitis B and C viruses, and influenza A and B viruses. The first experimental antivirals were developed in the 1960s. Interferons inhibit viral synthesis in infected cells. Almost all anti-microbials, including anti-virals, are subject to drug resistance as the pathogens mutate over time, becoming less susceptible to the treatment.

Viruses by themselves are not alive. They cannot grow or multiply on their own and need to enter a human or animal cell and take over the cell to help them multiply. An infected cell will produce viral particles instead of its usual products. They must first attach to a receptor on the cell surface. Each virus has its specific receptor. Viruses do not have the chemical machinery needed to survive on their own. They, thus seek out host cells in which they can multiply.

A cold or flu virus, for example, will target cells that line the respiratory or digestive tracts. The HIV (human immunodeficiency virus) that causes AIDS attacks the T-cells (a type of white blood cell that fights infection and disease) of the immune system. There are a few basic steps that all infecting viruses follow. These include: a virus particle attaches to a host cell. This is called the process of adsorption. The particle injects its DNA or RNA into the host cell. The invading DNA or RNA takes over the cell. The cellular enzymes start making new virus particles. The particles of the virus created by the infected cell, come together to form new viruses. The new viruses kill the host cell and break free and search for a new host cell.

Like antibiotics for bacteria, specific antivirals are used for specific viruses. Unlike most antibiotics, antiviral drugs do not destroy their target pathogen; instead they inhibit their development. Most of the antiviral drugs now available are designed to help deal with HIV, herpes viruses, the hepatitis B and C viruses, and influenza A and B viruses.

The antiviral drugs can alter the structure and genetic material of the invaded cell so the viruses can no longer use it to multiply. Sometimes the cell can work as normal after the viruses have left. Another method to prevent viruses multiplying is block enzyme activity in the invaded cell. Another method is by using interferon substances, produced by the virus-infected cells, to protect those that have not yet been invaded. By means of genetic engineering, interferon substances can be produced artificially.

Vaccines are probably the most successful method of dealing with viruses. By injecting weaker forms of the disease into the body, the body becomes immune to far deadlier diseases such as smallpox. If none of the above methods work, it is often left to the body's immune system to battle viral infection.

All viruses have a basic core consisting of nucleic acid and a shell, or capsid, made up of proteins. Viruses work by invading cells, making copies of themselves, and often destroying the invaded cell in the process. Viruses can work in many ways, including disrupting the functions of the cell while it is invaded. When they interact with the chromosomes in the invaded cell, they can cause cancer. Some viruses attack the immune system of the cell, causing widespread loss of immune system functions throughout the body.

A virus is composed of a strand of DNA or RNA encased in an envelope of protein, called a capsid. Because of their unique structure and method of causing disease, viruses cannot be treated with antibiotic drugs. How a virus infects a host is crucial to understanding how infections begin after individual virus particles infiltrate the host's cells. This can be accomplished because viruses are so tiny that they may slip through cellular defenses unopposed. Once inside a host cell, a virus moves to the cell's nucleus where all the DNA and RNA functions as instructions for the cell's operation. By inserting its own genetic information into the cell's nucleus a virus can hijack its function, causing it to produce and release more virus particles so the infection spreads. Another common effect of this cellular hijacking is the damage, breakdown and eventual death of the cell itself.

Like most drugs used to treat infectious pathogens, antivirals are targeted to specific strains of viruses and work in a variety of ways. Most antiviral drugs don't actually kill the virus particles themselves as inhibit their reproduction. Since viruses cannot reproduce without infecting a host cell, antiviral drugs have been designed to interfere with the infection process.

This interference may be achieved in numerous ways, including blocking the virus from the host cell, preventing the virus from releasing its genetic material once it reaches the nucleus and preventing the virus's genetic data from being spliced into the host cell's DNA. Various highly specific antiviral drugs have also been developed that target the enzymes and proteins that an infected host cell uses to assemble new virus particles and prevent them from functioning correctly. Such drugs must be designed very carefully so that they do not interfere with the metabolism of healthy cells. A final type of antiviral drug targets the virus indirectly, by increasing the efficiency with which the host's immune system can fight the viral infection.

Antiviral drugs are prescription medicines (pills, liquid, an inhaled powder, or an intravenous solution) that fight against the flu in your body. Antiviral drugs are not sold over-the-counter. You can only get them if you have a prescription from your doctor or health care provider. Antiviral drugs are different from antibiotics, which fight against bacterial infections.

Antiviral drugs are a second line of defense to treat the flu. A flu vaccine is still the first and best way to prevent influenza. When used for treatment, antiviral drugs can lessen symptoms and shorten the time you are sick by 1 or 2 days. They also can prevent serious flu complications, like pneumonia. For people with a high-risk medical condition, treatment with an antiviral drug can mean the difference between having milder illness instead of very serious illness that could result in a hospital stay.

Some side effects have been associated with the use of flu antiviral drugs, including nausea, vomiting, dizziness, runny or stuffy nose, cough, diarrhea, headache and some behavioral side effects. To treat the flu, Tamiflu and Relenza are usually prescribed for 5 days, although people hospitalized with the flu may need the medicine for longer than 5 days. Rapivab is administered intravenously for 15 to 30 minutes.

Following is a list of health and age factors that are known to increase a person's risk of getting serious complications from the flu: asthma, neurological and neurodevelopmental conditions, blood disorders (such as sickle cell disease), chronic lung disease, diabetes mellitus, heart disease, coronary artery disease, kidney disorders, liver disorders, metabolic disorders, morbid obesity, weakened immune system due to disease or medication or cancer, or those on chronic steroids.

Other people with high risk from the flu: adults 65 years and older, children younger than 5 years old, but especially children younger than 2 years old, pregnant women and women up to two weeks after the end of pregnancy, American Indians and Alaska Natives.

Certain antiviral medicines prevent the virus that causes shingles from multiplying. These medicines shorten the period of rash, reduce pain during the active stage of the illness, and reduce the chance of getting complications of shingles, such as post herpetic neuralgia. Antivirals may be taken orally or injected intravenously. Anyone who has shingles can use antivirals, but antivirals are particularly beneficial for adults older than 50 and people who have weak immune systems. They are also used for people who have severe rash and those who have a rash near an eye and/or on the forehead.

Antiviral medications may reduce the severity of shingles and speed healing. When acyclovir, famciclovir, or valacyclovir is taken within three days of getting shingles, these medicines can significantly reduce the duration of pain associated with shingles. These medicines also reduce the pain caused by post herpetic neuralgia.

The recent AIDS crisis is one of the most deadly in the world. The virus that causes AIDS, HIV, works like some other viruses in that it attacks the immune system of the cell, binding to the receptor proteins on some white blood cells, causing the entire immune system of the body to stop working. AIDS (Acquired Immunodeficiency Syndrome) refers to the immune system being completely deficient; so various opportunistic infections, of which there are 26, start to rapidly take effect. It is these diseases, or cancers that develop, that usually result in death, since that body cannot adequately defend itself.

Almost all anti-microbials, including anti-virals, are subject to drug resistance as the pathogens mutate over time, becoming less susceptible to the treatment. Although a course of antivirals can help prevent the flu, it is considered to be a far less effective prophylactic option than getting a dose of flu vaccine. In addition, physicians are reluctant to overprescribe antiviral drugs because this can lead to the appearance of drug-resistant flu viruses that are difficult to treat. Flu vaccines are available for each flu season from local health providers. Because the type A influenza mutates rapidly, a new form of the flu vaccine must be developed each year to protect people from the strains that experts believe will be most likely during that flu season.

Vaccines are usually derived from the very germs the vaccine is designed to protect against. A vaccine typically contains an agent that resembles a disease-causing microorganism, and is often made from weakened or killed forms of the microbe. The agent stimulates the body's immune system to recognize the agent as foreign, destroy it, and remember it, so that the immune system can more easily recognize and destroy any of these microorganisms that it later encounters.

Vaccines are of different types-live and attenuated, inactivated subunit, toxoid, conjugate, DNA, recombinant vector vaccines and other experimental vaccines. The earliest reports of vaccines seem to have originated from India and China in the 17th century and recorded in Ayurveda texts. The first description of a successful vaccination procedure came from Dr. Emmanuel Timoni in 1724, followed by Edward Jenner's independent description, half a century later, of a method for vaccinating humans against small pox. This technique was further developed by Louis Pasteur during the 19th century to produce vaccines against anthrax and rabies. Since then attempts have been made to develop more vaccines against many more diseases.

Live, attenuated vaccines are weakened microbes that help cause lifelong immunity by eliciting a strong immune response. A huge disadvantage of this type of vaccine is that because the virus is live, it can mutate and cause severe reactions in people with a weak immune system. Another limitation of this vaccine is that it has to be refrigerated to stay potent. Examples for this type include vaccines against chicken pox, measles and mumps.

Inactivated vaccines are dead microbes and safer than the former type, though these illicit a weaker immune response, and often have to be followed by booster shots. The DTap and Tdap vaccines are inactivated vaccines.

Antibiotics are usually given orally, intravenously or topically. The course may last from a minimum of 3-5 days or longer depending on the type and severity of the infection.

A large number of vaccines and their booster shots are usually scheduled before the age of two for children. In the United States, routine vaccinations for children include those against hepatitis A, B, polio, mumps, measles, rubella, diphtheria, pertussis, tetanus, chickenpox, rotavirus, influenza, meningococcal disease and pneumonia. This routine might differ in other countries and is continually being updated. Vaccinations for other infections such as shingles, HPV are also available. Though antibiotics are not considered unsafe, these compounds may cause certain adverse reactions. These include, fever, nausea, diarrhea and allergic reactions.

The CDC maintains that vaccines now produced meet very high safety standards so that the overall benefit and protection vaccines offer against diseases far outweighs any adverse reactions it might have in some individuals.

Because antibiotics are used a lot (and sometimes are used inappropriately) antibiotic resistance is becoming a common problem. It occurs when bacteria in your body change so that antibiotics don't work effectively to fight them anymore. This can happen when bacteria are repeatedly exposed to the same antibiotics or when bacteria are left in your body after you have been taking an antibiotic (such as when someone does not take the full course of their antibiotic medicine). These bacteria can multiply and become strong enough to resist the antibiotic in the future. Antibiotics are not needed for and won't work against viral infections such as a cold, the flu (influenza). Antibiotics help treat illnesses that are caused by bacteria, certain parasites and some types of fungus. Simply put, antibiotics cannot kill viruses because viruses have different structures and replicate in a different way than bacteria. Overuse of antibiotics on the other hand has led to superbugs, and now bacterial resistance is on the rise. Vaccines stimulate your own immune system to produce antibodies, which then go out and recognize the virus to inactivate it before it can cause disease.

Why won't my medication work?

1. Most drugs are manufactured for a specific ailment. If your diagnosis is wrong, and if you were prescribed a specific drug for a disease, you will not receive any relief.

2. Your prescribed drug may be adversely affected by your hormones.

3. Other drugs that you are taking may interfere with your medicine. Drug-drug interactions occur when two or more drugs react with each other. Drug-food/beverage interactions result from drugs reacting with foods or beverages. Drug-

condition interactions may occur when an existing medical condition makes certain drugs potentially harmful

4. Your drug won't work if it is not absorbed by your stomach or small intestine due to excess acid in your gut.

5. Many drugs will not work unless the drug is converted into a new medication in your liver. You may have a genetic mutation which prevents this conversion.

6. Your dose of medication may not be sufficient.

7. Your medicine may not be potent enough.

8. Most drugs need to be absorbed from your stomach or small intestine to enter your blood stream. Abdominal surgery may not leave a way for a drug to get into your blood stream.

9. Your liver may filter a large portion of the drug before it gets to the proper receptor.

10. Your kidneys may excrete your drug too quickly before it has time to give you relief.

11. Some foods that you eat may interact with your medication causing your medication not to work.

12. Smoking may inhibit the effects of some medications.

13. Many medications are divided into subclasses. A change from one subclass to another subclass may be effective for your condition.

14. Other factors can affect how quickly a drug is absorbed. For example, most absorption of oral drugs occurs in the small intestine. If a patient has had large sections of the small intestine surgically removed, drug absorption decreases. If your body does not absorb enough drug, it may not work.

15. Pain and stress can also decrease the amount of drug absorbed by your body.

16. Drug tolerance occurs when a patient develops a decreased response to a drug over time. You then require a larger dose of medication to produce the same response.

17. Some generic drugs may not work as well as the brand name drugs.

18. Your gender may affect how your drug works.

19. Medications may be given by mouth, by patch, by suppository, by injection or by nasal spray. If one form of drug is ineffective another form may work.

20. Some drugs compete for the same receptor (e.g. Narcan and Morphine where Narcan pushes the Morphine off the mu receptor which stops the effects of the Morphine).

21. You must read all the instructions and warnings that come with your medication for your drug to work effectively.

Interactions between alcohol and certain antibiotics may occur and may cause side effects and decreased effectiveness of antibiotic therapy. The standard protocol followed by most doctors is to prescribe a general or broad-spectrum antibiotic for an infection and see if it works. If it doesn't work, doctors often resort to a trial and error process in the hope of eventually finding an effective drug. Antibacterial-resistant strains and species now contribute to the emergence of diseases that were for a while well controlled. Widespread usage of antibiotics in hospitals has also been associated with increases in bacterial strains and species that no longer respond to treatment with the most common antibiotics. Some foods, supplements and medications can interact or make antibiotics less effective. Antibiotic resistance is harmful. As more antibiotics are introduced into our environment, by either over-prescribing or entering our food chain through their use in the dairy, poultry, and livestock industries, more strains of bacteria have the potential to become resistant.

## 26. Hormones

A hormone is any member of a class of signaling molecules produced by endocrine glands. Endocrine glands, which are special groups of cells, make hormones. The major endocrine glands are the pituitary, pineal, thymus, thyroid, adrenal glands, and pancreas. This chapter will discuss growth hormone, estrogen, progesterone, testosterone and DHEA. Hormones are used to communicate between organs and tissues to regulate physiological and behavioral activities, such as digestion, metabolism, respiration, tissue function, sensory perception, sleep, excretion, lactation, stress, growth and development, movement, reproduction, and mood are thus readily transported through the circulatory system. Hormones have the following effects on the body: stimulation or inhibition of growth, wake-sleep cycle and other circadian rhythms, mood swings, suppression of activation or inhibition of the immune system, regulation of metabolism, preparation of the body for mating, fighting, fleeing, and other activities, preparation of the body for a new phase of life, such as puberty, parenting, and menopause, control of the reproductive cycle, hunger cravings or sexual arousal.

Luteinizing hormone, follicle-stimulating hormone and thyroid-stimulating hormone are examples of glycoprotein hormones Eicosanoids hormones are derived from lipids such as arachidonic acid, lipoxins and prostaglandins, and steroid hormones, which include the sex hormones estradiol and testosterone as well as the stress hormone cortisol.

Vertebrate hormones fall into four main chemical classes: amino acid derived, which include melatonin and thyroxine, polypeptides and proteins. Examples of protein hormones include insulin and growth hormone. More complex protein hormones bear carbohydrate side-chains and are called glycoprotein hormones.

Growth hormone treatment refers to the use of growth hormone (GH) as a prescription medication. It has been recommended that adult patients diagnosed with growth hormone deficiency be administered an individualized GH treatment regimen. Benefits include improved bone density increased muscle mass, decrease of adipose tissue, faster hair and nail growth, strengthened immune system, increased circulatory system, and improved blood lipid levels. Growth hormone available in the U.S. included: Nutropin, Humatrope, Genotropin, Norditropin, Tev-Tropin and Saizen.

In adults, the approved uses of GH include: short bowel syndrome, a condition in which nutrients are not properly absorbed due to severe intestinal disease or the surgical removal of a large portion of the small intestine, GH deficiency due to

WHY WON'T MY MECIDICATION WORK? 237

rare pituitary tumors or their treatment, and muscle-wasting disease associated with HIV/AIDS. Because the body's GH levels naturally decrease with age, some so-called anti-aging experts have speculated and claimed that GH products could reverse age-related bodily deterioration. GH can also increase the risk of diabetes and contribute to the growth of cancerous tumors.

 Dehydroepiandrosterone (DHEA) is a hormone that is naturally made by the human body. It can be made in the laboratory from chemicals found in wild yam and soy. DHEA is used for slowing or reversing, aging, improving thinking skills in older people, and slowing the progress of Alzheimer's disease. DHEA is being investigated and may eventually be approved by the Food and Drug Administration as a prescription drug for treating systemic lupus erythematosus and improving bone mineral density in women with lupus who are taking steroid drugs for treatment.  is a hormone that comes from the adrenal gland. It is also made in the brain. DHEA leads to the production of androgens and estrogens (male and female sex hormones). DHEA levels in your body begin to decrease after age 30. Levels decrease more quickly in women. Lower DHEA levels are found in people with hormonal disorders, HIV/AIDS, Alzheimer's disease, heart disease, depression, diabetes, inflammation, immune disorders, and osteoporosis. Some patients try DHEA to treat osteoporosis, multiple sclerosis and low levels of steroid hormones, chronic fatigue syndrome and to slow the progression of Parkinson's disease. DHEA may stimulate tumor growth in types of cancer that are sensitive to hormones, such as some types of breast, uterine, and prostate cancer. DHEA may also increase prostate swelling in men with an enlarged prostate gland. DHEA supplements may also raise the risk of diabetes and stroke.

Corticosteroids, birth control taken by mouth, and agents that treat psychiatric disorders may reduce DHEA levels. Lower DHEA levels are found in people with hormonal disorders, HIV/AIDS, Alzheimer's disease, heart disease, depression, diabetes, inflammation, immune disorders, and osteoporosis. DHEA is a steroid hormone. High doses may cause aggressiveness, irritability, trouble sleeping, and the growth of body or facial hair on women. DHEA should not be used with tamoxifen, as it may promote tamoxifen resistance. DHEA is readily available in the United States, and is marketed as an over-the-counter dietary supplement. DHEA supplementation in elderly men can induce a small but significant positive effect on body composition that is strictly dependent on DHEA conversion into its bioactive metabolites such as androgens or estrogens.

Testosterone is a steroid hormone and is found in humans and other vertebrates. In humans and other mammals, testosterone is secreted primarily by the testicles of males and, to a lesser extent, the ovaries of females. In men, testosterone plays a key role in the development of male reproductive tissues such as the testis and prostate as well as promoting secondary sexual characteristics such as increased muscle, bone mass, and the growth of body hair. A number of lawsuits are currently underway against testosterone manufacturers, alleging a significantly increased rate of stroke and heart attack in elderly men who use testosterone supplements.

That explosion in testosterone use has occurred despite a lack of evidence showing it is effective. The surge has been attributed to an aggressive marketing campaign by manufacturers alerting men to the potential effects of low T, such as fatigue, sexual dysfunction, declining muscle mass and gains in body fat.

The benefits and risks of testosterone therapy have not been established for the treatment of men who have low testosterone levels due to aging, even if there are symptoms that seem related to the low testosterone. Testosterone supplements increase a man's risk of heart attack or stroke. These supplements are unlikely to do much for most men whose testosterone dips solely due to age.

On average, menopause occurs at age 51. When it does, a woman's body produces less estrogen and progesterone. The drop of estrogen levels at menopause can cause uncomfortable symptoms, including: hot flashes night sweats vaginal dryness or itching and loss of libido or sex drive.

Lower levels of estrogen may also increase a woman's risk for heart disease, stroke, osteoporosis and fractures. If your body produces too much testosterone, you may have irregular or absent menstrual periods. You may also have more body hair than the average woman. At menopause, estrogen levels fall to very low levels. Interestingly, taking oral estrogen does not improve depression in women after menopause. Estrogens mimic the physiologic effects of naturally occurring female sex hormones. Estrogens are used to correct estrogen deficient states and, along with hormonal contraceptives, prevent pregnancy. Estrogens are prescribed: primarily for hormone replacement therapy in postmenopausal women to relieve symptoms caused by loss of ovarian function, for hormonal replacement therapy in women with primary ovarian failure or for prevention and treatment of osteoporosis in postmenopausal women, and in patients who have undergone surgical castration and palliatively to treat advanced, inoperable breast cancer in post-menopausal women.

Most hormones initiate a cellular response by initially binding to either cell membrane associated or intracellular receptors. A cell may have several different receptor types that recognize the same hormone but activate different signal transduction pathways, or a cell may have several different receptors that recognize different hormones and activate the same biochemical pathway.

Oral hormones are less effective because anything taken orally will be subject to the filtering organs, resulting in less bioavailability than the transdermal delivery methods. Reports state that over 80% of the hormone used in oral methods is filtered by the liver. Women take progesterone by mouth for inducing menstrual periods; and treating abnormal uterine bleeding associated with hormonal imbalance, and severe symptoms of premenstrual syndrome (PMS). Progesterone is also used in combination with the hormone estrogen to oppose estrogen as part of hormone-replacement therapy. If estrogen is given without progesterone, estrogen increases the risk of uterine cancer. Progesterone is also used to ease withdrawal symptoms when certain drugs (Valium like drugs) are discontinued.

Common side effects of progesterone include: headaches, painful or tender breasts, stomach pain, dizziness and depression. Side Effects of progesterone include: dementia in post-menopausal women who are more than 65 years of age, vomiting, swelling in the feet, ankles, and lower legs, blood clots, heart attacks, stroke, or blood clots in the lungs, missed periods or breakthrough bleeding and breast cancer. Transdermal delivery of progesterone is the preferred method for supplementing with the use of natural progesterone. The skin is the largest vital organ in the human body.

Why won't my medication work?

In general, medications may not work for the following reasons:

1. Most drugs are manufactured for a specific ailment. If your diagnosis is wrong, and if you were prescribed a specific drug for a disease, you will not receive any relief.

2. Your prescribed drug may be adversely affected by your hormones.

3. Other drugs that you are taking may interfere with your medicine. Drug-drug interactions occur when two or more drugs react with each other. Drug-food/beverage interactions result from drugs reacting with foods or beverages. Drug-condition interactions may occur when an existing medical condition makes certain drugs potentially harmful

4. Your drug won't work if it is not absorbed by your stomach or small intestine due to excess acid in your gut.

5. Many drugs will not work unless the drug is converted into a new medication in your liver. You may have a genetic mutation which prevents this conversion.

6. Your dose of medication may not be sufficient.

7. Your medicine may not be potent enough.

8. Most drugs need to be absorbed from your stomach or small intestine to enter your blood stream. Abdominal surgery may not leave a way for a drug to get into your blood stream.

9. Your liver may filter a large portion of the drug before it gets to the proper receptor.

10. Your kidneys may excrete your drug too quickly before it has time to give you relief.

11. Some foods that you eat may interact with your medication causing your medication not to work.

12. Smoking may inhibit the effects of some medications.

13. Many medications are divided into subclasses. A change from one subclass to another subclass may be effective for your condition.

14. Other factors can affect how quickly a drug is absorbed. For example, most absorption of oral drugs occurs in the small intestine. If a patient has had large sections of the small intestine surgically removed, drug absorption decreases. If your body does not absorb enough drug, it may not work.

15. Pain and stress can also decrease the amount of drug absorbed by your body.

16. Drug tolerance occurs when a patient develops a decreased response to a drug over time. You then require a larger dose of medication to produce the same response.

17. Some generic drugs may not work as well as the brand name drugs.

18. Your gender may affect how your drug works.

19. Medications may be given by mouth, by patch, by suppository, by injection or by nasal spray. If one form of drug is ineffective another form may work.

20. Some drugs compete for the same receptor (e.g. Narcan and Morphine where Narcan pushes the Morphine off the mu receptor which stops the effects of the Morphine).

21. You must read all the instructions and warnings that come with your medication for your drug to be effective.

Hormones are powerful. Your hormone may not work if the amount that you take is insufficient. It takes only a small amount to cause vast fluctuations in your cells or your entire body. That is why too much or too little of a certain hormone can be serious. Laboratory tests can measure your hormone levels. Your health care provider may perform these tests if you have symptoms of a hormone disorder.

## 27. Erectile Dysfunction Drugs

Seventeen per cent of men between 18 and 55 experience occasional impotence, while 6% have regular erectile difficulties. For men over 55, that number increases to one in three. Some common causes of impotence are diabetes, heart disease, and psychological problems. It also frequently occurs after prostate cancer surgery.

Because Viagra works in a way that's similar to drugs that contain nitrates, however, it isn't recommended for men who take nitrates for heart disease or those with certain other heart conditions. In some men, it causes bad headaches. In others, it doesn't work. In some instances, men may notice they have trouble telling blue and green colors apart when they start taking the drug.

Oral medications are often the first line of treatment for erectile dysfunction. For most men who have trouble keeping an erection firm enough for sex, these medications work well and cause few side effects. Sildenafil (Viagra), vardenafil (Levitra, Staxyn), tadalafil (Cialis) and avanafil (Stendra) are oral medications that reverse erectile dysfunction by enhancing the effects of nitric oxide, a natural chemical your body produces that relaxes muscles in the penis. This increases blood flow and allows you to get an erection in response to sexual stimulation.

Although they work in similar ways, each oral medication has a slightly different chemical makeup. These minor differences affect the way each medication works, such as how quickly it takes effect and wears off, and the potential side effects. Your doctor will consider these factors as well as any health problems you have and possible interactions with other medications you take.

Medications for erectile dysfunction might not work or might be dangerous if you: take nitrate drugs commonly prescribed for chest pain such as nitroglycerin, isosorbide mononitrate and isosorbide dinitrate, have very low blood pressure (hypotension) or uncontrolled high blood pressure (hypertension), have severe liver disease, or have kidney disease that requires dialysis.

Sildenafil (Viagra). is most effective when taken on an empty stomach one hour before sex. It is effective for up to six hours. Vardenafil (Levitra) also is most effective when taken one hour before sex and can be taken with or without food. It's effective for up to seven hours. Tadalafil (Cialis) is taken with or without food about one to two hours before sex. It's effective for 36 hours. It can be taken in a small dose daily or in a larger dose as needed. Avanafil (Stendra) is taken with or without food 15 to 30 minutes before sex, depending on the dose. It lasts up to six hours.

During an erection, blood flows quickly into the penis, which increases its length, width, and firmness. If the arteries are too narrow or if blood drains too quickly through the veins, men may have trouble achieving or maintaining an erection. If you are troubled by occasional erectile dysfunction, remember that arousal takes longer as you get older and that satisfaction should not be equated with performance.

Make sure you're getting the right treatment for any health conditions that could be causing or worsening your erectile dysfunction. Medications for erectile dysfunction might not work or might be dangerous if you: Take nitrate drugs commonly prescribed for chest pain (angina) such as nitroglycerin, isosorbide mononitrate and isosorbide dinitrate, have very low blood pressure (hypotension) or uncontrolled high blood pressure (hypertension), have severe liver disease or kidney disease that requires dialysis, take anti-depressants and nicotine. Psychological causes include performance anxiety as well as stress, and mental disorders. Aging is another cause, and erectile dysfunction is four times more common in men their 60s than those in their 40s. Kidney failure and diseases such as diabetes mellitus and multiple sclerosis are also associated with erectile dysfunction.

In general, your medications may not work for the following reasons:

1. Most drugs are manufactured for a specific ailment. If your diagnosis is wrong, and if you were prescribed a specific drug for a disease, you will not receive any relief.

2. Your prescribed drug may be adversely affected by your hormones.

3. Other drugs that you are taking may interfere with your medicine. Drug-drug interactions occur when two or more drugs react with each other. Drug-food/beverage interactions result from drugs reacting with foods or beverages. Drug-condition interactions may occur when an existing medical condition makes certain drugs potentially harmful.

4. Your drug won't work if it is not absorbed by your stomach or small intestine due to excess acid in your gut.

5. Many drugs will not work unless the drug is converted into a new medication in your liver. You may have a genetic mutation which prevents this conversion.

6. Your dose of medication may not be sufficient.

7. Your medicine may not be potent enough.

8. Most drugs need to be absorbed from your stomach or small intestine to enter your blood stream. Abdominal surgery may not leave a way for a drug to get into your blood stream.

9. Your liver may filter a large portion of the drug before it gets to the proper receptor.

## WHY WON'T MY MECIDICATION WORK? 249

10. Your kidneys may excrete your drug too quickly before it has time to give you relief.

11. Some foods that you eat may interact with your medication causing your medication not to work.

12. Smoking may inhibit the effects of some medications.

13. Many medications are divided into subclasses. A change from one subclass to another subclass may be effective for your condition.

14. Other factors can affect how quickly a drug is absorbed. For example, most absorption of oral drugs occurs in the small intestine. If a patient has had large sections of the small intestine surgically removed, drug absorption decreases. If your body does not absorb enough drug, it may not work.

15. Pain and stress can also decrease the amount of drug absorbed by your body.

16. Drug tolerance occurs when a patient develops a decreased response to a drug over time. You then require a larger dose of medication to produce the same response.

17. Some generic drugs may not work as well as the brand name drugs.

18. Your gender may affect how your drug works.

19. Medications may be given by mouth, by patch, by suppository, by injection or by nasal spray. If one form of drug is ineffective another form may work.

20. Some drugs compete for the same receptor (e.g. Narcan and Morphine where Narcan pushes the Morphine off the mu receptor which stops the effects of the Morphine).

21. You must read all the instructions and warnings that come with your medication for your drug to work effectively.

An ED drug will not work if the arterial blood inflow is caused by the arteries which are too narrow. The cause of erectile dysfunction in men with diabetes is usually related to a decrease in the blood supply to the penis as well as to injury to the nerves that are responsible for the erection mechanism. A decrease in testosterone production has also been identified as the cause of ED in some men with diabetes. Another reason for the drugs not to work as intended is the consumption of a high-fat meal before or along with taking the drug because the fat in a meal can decrease absorption of the ED medicine from the gastrointestinal tract. Before a patient concludes that oral drugs don't work the patient should have his testosterone level checked to rule out hormone deficiency as the cause of his sexual dysfunction.

Diabetes, high-cholesterol levels, high blood pressure, and smoking contribute to atherosclerosis and therefore to ED. If oral medications do not work, the next step for most men would be a trial of intraurethral prostaglandin. This is a suppository that is inserted by the patient into the urethral meatus; approximately 30 minutes before intercourse is anticipated. It is easy for most men to learn how to use the medication, and it works well with a good result in 30% to 60% of patients who fail oral medications. The medication is safe. If prostaglandin administered intraurethrally is not effective, various vacuum suction devices are available that should work.

## 28. Muscle Relaxants

The skeletal muscle relaxants are a diverse set of drugs that are used for treating muscle spasticity or spasms, which can cause pain and interfere with your functional ability. A muscle relaxant is a drug which affects skeletal muscle function and decreases the muscle tone. It may be used to alleviate symptoms such as muscle spasms, pain, and hyperreflexia. Spasticity, or having stiff, rigid muscles with exaggerated reflexes, generally lasts a long time. It arises from conditions affecting the brain and/or spinal cord, such as cerebral palsy, multiple sclerosis, and stroke. Muscle spasms, on the other hand, are usually temporary and are associated with conditions affecting the muscles, bones, and associated structures, such as tension headaches, back or neck pain, and fibromyalgia. Muscle relaxants are used to reduce muscle tone and relax muscles, treating symptoms for pain and muscle spasms.

Muscle relaxants such are commonly prescribed for low back pain or neck pain, fibromyalgia, tension headaches and the myofascial pain syndrome. In general, no high-quality evidence supports their use in these syndromes. Muscle relaxants are thought to be useful in painful disorders based on the theory that pain induces spasm and spasm causes pain. However, considerable evidence contradicts this theory. Muscle relaxants are not approved by FDA for long-term use. Patients most commonly report sedation as the main adverse effect of muscle relaxants.

The muscle relaxants in current use have variable mechanisms of action, efficacy and adverse effects. This type of medications is well tolerated, with the most common side effects being drowsiness and nausea. The latency of the liver injury is variable. Large spinal cord nerves control skeletal muscles. The nerve cells projections go outward to join with muscle cells. The neuromuscular junction is where the muscle and nerve connect. Here a chemical known as a neurotransmitter is released that runs across the area between the muscle and the nerve, causing the desired response. The neurotransmitters glycine and GABA reduce muscle activity, while acetylcholine stimulates muscle activity.

The majority of the published clinical trials evaluating the safety of muscle relaxants do not mention hepatotoxicity or aminotransferase elevations. Rare cases of drug-induced jaundice have occurred with some but not all the muscle relaxants. Agents that have been fairly clearly linked to clinically apparent acute liver injury include chlorzoxazone, dantrolene, quinine and tizanidine. Cases of acute liver failure and death have been reported after chlorzoxazone and dantrolene therapy. There is little evidence to suggest that baclofen, carisoprodol, cyclobenzaprine, metaxalone, methocarbamol or orphenadrine is associated with significant liver injury, and if it occurs, hepatotoxicity from these agents must be exceedingly rare.

Baclofen is a gamma-amino butyric acid (GABA) derivative that acts as an agonist to the GABA B receptor thereby activating potassium channels and reducing calcium conductance leading to hypotonia and muscle relaxation. Baclofen acts primarily at the level of the spinal cord, inhibiting synaptic reflexes. Baclofen reduces the number and severity of muscle spasms and relieves pain, clonus and muscle rigidity due to spasticity. Baclofen is indicated primarily for treatment of spasticity from spinal cord injuries and multiple sclerosis. It has been used off label as adjunctive therapy to help with alcohol abstinence and withdrawal.

Baclofen was approved for use in the United States in 1977 and is widely used with more than 3 million prescriptions filled yearly. Baclofen is available in various generic forms as well as under the brand names of Lioresal and Remular in tablets of 10 or 20 mg and in formulations for intrathecal injections of 0.5 mg/mL. The recommended adult dose for spasticity is 10 to 20 mg orally three to four times daily. The dose should be increased and tapered gradually. The most common side effects of baclofen are nausea, drowsiness, confusion, dizziness and fatigue.

Carisoprodol is a carbamate derivative similar to meprobamate. Its mechanism of action as a muscle relaxant is unknown, but it is a sedative and may act centrally by modifying perception of pain without affecting pain reflexes. Carisoprodol is recommended for treatment of acute, painful disorders of the musculoskeletal system. Carisoprodol is available in 250 and 350 mg tablets in generic formulations and under the trade names of Soma, Carisoma, Sodol and Vanadom. Fixed combinations of carisoprodol with aspirin or codeine are also attainable. The recommended adult dosage is 250 to 350 mg three to four times daily for 2 to 3 weeks. Carisoprodol was approved for use in the United States in 1959 and is widely used with more than 10 million prescriptions filled yearly. It is available by prescription only and is classified as a Schedule IV agent, meaning that it has a low potential for abuse and physical or psychological dependence and has an accepted medical usefulness. Common side effects include dizziness, drowsiness and headache. Overdose can cause progressive obtundation, coma, neuromuscular rigidity, myoclonus and seizures.

Chlorzoxazone acts centrally rather than directly on muscles to relieve muscle spasms, either through its sedative effects or other unknown mechanisms. Chlorzoxazone is indicated for therapy of low back pain and muscle spasms, although its overall efficacy is considered only fair. Chlorzoxazone was

# WHY WON'T MY MECIDICATION WORK? 257

approved for use in the United States in 1958 and is still widely used. It is available in various generic forms as well as under the brand names of Parafon Forte and Remular in tablets of 250 or 500 mg. The usual recommended dose in adults is 250-750 mg orally three to four times daily reducing the dose to the lowest effective level once a response occurs. Chlorzoxazone is typically given for 1 to 4 weeks only. Common side effects of chlorzoxazone include dizziness, drowsiness, headache, fatigue and tremor.

Cyclobenzaprine is a tricyclic anti-depressant derivative that relaxes the skeletal muscles by an unknown mechanism of action. Cyclobenzaprine is also a central nervous system depressant, and its efficacy may be related to its sedative effects. Cyclobenzaprine is used for the treatment of painful muscle spasms from acute muscle conditions. The recommended dosage in adults is 5 to 10 mg three times daily for 3 to 4 weeks. Cyclobenzaprine is available in tablets of 5 and 10 mg in multiple generic forms and under the trade names of Flexeril, Flexamid and Amrix. Extended release capsules of 15 and 30 mg are also available.

Cyclobenzaprine was approved for use in the United States in 1977, and it remains widely used with more than 18 million prescriptions filled year. It is usually administered for limited periods of time. Common side effects include sleepiness, dry mouth, dizziness and headache.

Dantrolene is a lipid soluble diphenylhydantoin analogue that inhibits muscle contractions by decreasing the release of calcium from the sarcoplasmic reticulum in target tissue. Dantrolene is used for the treatment of chronic spasticity and treatment for and prophylaxis against malignant hyperthermia (based upon its ability to block calcium release, which is the initiating event in malignant hyperthermia).

In adults, the recommended initial dose for spasticity is 25 mg daily with subsequent increases to a dose of 25 to 100 mg three times daily. Dantrolene is also available in parenteral formulations for therapy of acute episodes of malignant hyperthermia; the recommended initial dose being 1 mg/kg intravenously. For prophylaxis against hyperthermia, dantrolene is given orally in doses of 4 to 8 mg/kg daily. Common side effects include weakness, nausea, drowsiness, fatigue and dizziness.

Metaxalone acts centrally as a skeletal muscle relaxant, but its efficacy and precise mechanism of action are not well documented. Metaxalone was approved for use in the United States in 1962, and it remains a widely used muscle relaxant. Current indications include the treatment of pain from acute musculoskeletal conditions and muscle spasms. The recommended dosage is 800 mg orally three to four times daily. Metaxalone is available by prescription only in 400 and 800 mg tablets in generic forms as well as under the commercial name Skelaxin. Sparse data are available regarding metaxalone safety. Side effects are not common but can include drowsiness, dizziness, headache, nausea, and dry mouth.

Methocarbamol is a guaifenesin derivative and acts centrally as a muscle relaxant by an unknown mechanism. Methocarbamol was approved for use in the United States in 1957, and currently more than 3 million prescriptions are filled yearly. Methocarbamol is indicated for the relief of acute, painful musculoskeletal conditions. Methocarbamol is available in 500 and 750 mg tablets in several generic formulations both alone and in combination with other drugs and under the brand names of Robaxin and Marbaxin. The recommended dosage is 1500 mg orally three to four times daily. The most common side effects of methocarbamol are drowsiness blurred vision, headache, nausea and skin rash.

Orphenadrine is a centrally acting, non-opiate analgesic and muscle relaxant. It is a methyl derivative of diphenhydramine (a commonly used anti-histamine), but its mechanism of action in causing analgesia and skeletal muscle relaxation is not well defined. Orphenadrine has anticholinergic activity and may act centrally on pain perception. Orphenadrine is currently used for the treatment of acute, painful musculoskeletal conditions and can be given orally or parenterally. Orphenadrine was approved for use as a muscle relaxant in the United States in 1957, and it is still in wide use. Orphenadrine is available in multiple generic forms as standard and extended release tablets of 100 mg. It is also available under commercial names such as Norgesic, Norflex, Deenar, Banflex, Disipal and X-Otag. The recommended dosage is 100 mg twice daily. Orphenadrine is also available in parenteral formulations under the names of Flexoject and Myolin. The parenteral dose recommendation is 60 mg either intravenously or intramuscularly twice daily. The most common side effects are those typical of anti-cholinergics including drowsiness, dry mouth, diaphoresis, flushing, confusion and visual disturbances. Orphenadrine also has a potential for abuse and fatal overdoses have been reported.

Tizanidine is an imidazoline derivative and is a centrally acting muscle relaxant used for therapy of acute muscle spasms and chronic spasticity. The mechanism by which tizanidine causes skeletal muscle relaxation is not well known; it appears to act at the level of spinal cord pain reflexes, most likely through activity as an alpha-adrenergic agonist in inhibiting activity of motor neurons. Tizanidine was approved for use in the United States in 1996, and currently several million prescriptions are filled yearly. The current indications are limited to short-term management of spasticity. Tizanidine is available in several generic forms as well as under the brand name of Zanaflex in tablets and capsules of 2, 4 or 6 mg. The recommended dose in adults is 2 to 6 mg orally three to four times daily. Common side effects include tiredness, drowsiness, dizziness, muscular weakness, dry mouth and occasionally hypotension.

In general, your medications may not work for the following reasons:

1. Most drugs are manufactured for a specific ailment. If your diagnosis is wrong, and if you were prescribed a specific drug for a disease, you will not receive any relief.

2. Your prescribed drug may be adversely affected by your hormones.

3. Other drugs that you are taking may interfere with your medicine. Drug-drug interactions occur when two or more drugs react with each other. Drug-food/beverage interactions result from drugs reacting with foods or beverages. Drug-condition interactions may occur when an existing medical condition makes certain drugs potentially harmful.

4. Your drug won't work if it is not absorbed by your stomach or small intestine due to excess acid in your gut.

5. Many drugs will not work unless the drug is converted into a new medication in your liver. You may have a genetic mutation which prevents this conversion.

6. Your dose of medication may not be sufficient.

7. Your medicine may not be potent enough.

8. Most drugs need to be absorbed from your stomach or small intestine to enter your blood stream. Abdominal surgery may not leave a way for a drug to get into your blood stream.

9. Your liver may filter a large portion of the drug before it gets to the proper receptor.

10. Your kidneys may excrete your drug too quickly before it has time to give you relief.

11. Some foods that you eat may interact with your medication causing your medication not to work.

12. Smoking may inhibit the effects of some medications.

13. Many medications are divided into subclasses. A change from one subclass to another subclass may be effective for your condition.

14. Other factors can affect how quickly a drug is absorbed. For example, most absorption of oral drugs occurs in the small intestine. If a patient has had large sections of the small intestine surgically removed, drug absorption decreases. If your body does not absorb enough drug, it may not work.

15. Pain and stress can also decrease the amount of drug absorbed by your body.

# WHY WON'T MY MECIDICATION WORK?

16. Drug tolerance occurs when a patient develops a decreased response to a drug over time. You then require a larger dose of medication to produce the same response.

17. Some generic drugs may not work as well as the brand name drugs.

18. Your gender may affect how your drug works.

19. Medications may be given by mouth, by patch, by suppository, by injection or by nasal spray. If one form of drug is ineffective another form may work.

20. Some drugs compete for the same receptor (e.g. Narcan and Morphine where Narcan pushes the Morphine off the mu receptor which stops the effects of the Morphine).

21. You must read all the instructions and warnings that come with your medication for your drug to work effectively.

Your muscle relaxant may not work unless you take it at the proper time. Muscle relaxant medicines work best when they are taken before bedtime. They should not be used by a person who needs to drive or operate machinery. Muscle relaxers and pain medications are designed to give patients relief from the symptoms they are experiencing. What needs to be addressed is the problem that has initially caused the pain. Muscle trigger point injections may stop the muscle pain if the medications do not work. They should not be used by a person who needs to drive or operate machinery. It is not that the pain medications and muscle relaxers don't work; they just don't cure the problem. Muscle relaxers and pain medications are designed to give patients relief from the symptoms they are experiencing. What needs to be addressed is the problem that has initially caused the pain. Muscle trigger point injections may stop the muscle pain if the medications do not work.

Limiting muscle spasms and improving range of motion will prepare a patient for therapeutic exercises, which will provide the patient with more lasting pain relief. Muscle spasm of local origin needs to be clinically differentiated from spasticity and sustained muscle contraction in the setting of the central nervous system and upper motor neuron injury.

## 29. Sleep Medications

Between a third and half of all Americans have insomnia and complain of poor sleep. Insomnia is the inability to fall asleep or to remain asleep long enough to feel rested, especially when this is a problem that continues over time. Patients may complain of difficulty getting to sleep or staying asleep, intermittent wakefulness during the night, early-morning awakening, or combinations of any of these. Transient episodes are usually of little significance. Stress, caffeine, physical discomfort, daytime napping, and early bedtimes are common factors. Psychiatric disorders are often associated with persistent insomnia. Heavy smoking (more than a pack a day) causes difficulty falling asleep.

There are two broad classes of treatment for insomnia, and the two may be combined: psychological and pharmacologic. In general, it is appropriate to use medications for short courses of 1-2 weeks. The medications described above have largely replaced barbiturates as hypnotic agents because of their greater safety in case of an overdose.

Sometimes prescription drugs used mainly to treat depression may ease insomnia when taken in lower doses. Although widely used, these are not approved by the Food and Drug Administration for insomnia only. When insomnia is secondary to depression or anxiety, antidepressants may improve both conditions at the same time. Examples include: amitriptyline or trazodone.

All sleep medications work on the brain to promote drowsiness. Some drugs are specially designed as sleep aids; others are medicines with sedation as a side effect. Diphenhydramine is an over-the-counter medicine commonly taken for allergy symptoms. One of its side effects is drowsiness, and for this reason, diphenhydramine is often used as a sleep aid. Many of the most popular over-the-counter sleep aids contain diphenhydramine.

Selective gamma-aminobutyric acid (GABA) medications are among the newest sleep medicines and include: Ambien (zolpidem tartrate), Ambien CR (zolpidem tartrate extended release), Lunesta (eszopiclone) and Sonata (zaleplon). These sleeping pills work on the GABA receptors in the brain, which help control our level of alertness or relaxation. Ambien and other medicines in this class have also been blamed for episodes of sleepwalking. Ramelteon (Rozerem) is the newest prescription sleep medicine, and ramelteon works well in older adults with chronic insomnia. Benzodiazepines are older medicines that effectively help people get to sleep. Physicians usually avoid these drugs because of the possibility for drug dependence.

To enhance sleep do the following: No caffeine later in the day. Avoid nicotine or alcohol two to three hours before bedtime. Use your bedroom only for sleeping and sex. Maintain a regular sleep-wake schedule on all days, including weekends. Exercise regularly but complete it several hours before bedtime. Finish eating at least 2-3 hours before bedtime. Create a restful sleep environment by reducing noise, light, and temperature extremes with ear plugs, window blinds, an electric blanket, or air conditioner.

Many sleep disorders are brought on by underlying physical problems, like obesity or emotional issues like depression. Xanax, Valium, Klonpin and Ativan are anti-anxiety medications and can increase drowsiness and help you sleep. All benzodiazepines are however, potentially addictive. However, sleeping pills that are benzodiazepines belong to a group of medicines called central nervous system depressants, which slow down the nervous system. The longer you use tranquilizers and sleeping pills the more anxious you become. In the beginning, they help you relax and fall asleep. But after a few months, they have the opposite effect.

The following are sleep medication examples that help you fall asleep but can also lead to dependence: triazolam (Halcion), zaleplon (Sonata) and zolpidem (Ambien). The following drugs help you fall asleep and stay asleep but can lead to dependence: eszopiclone (Lunesta), temazepam (Restoril), and zolpidem (Ambien).

In general, your medications may not work for the following reasons:

1. Most drugs are manufactured for a specific ailment. If your diagnosis is wrong, and if you were prescribed a specific drug for a disease, you will not receive any relief.

2. Your prescribed drug may be adversely affected by your hormones.

3. Other drugs that you are taking may interfere with your medicine. Drug-drug interactions occur when two or more drugs react with each other. Drug-food/beverage interactions result from drugs reacting with foods or beverages. Drug-condition interactions may occur when an existing medical condition makes certain drugs potentially harmful.

4. Your drug won't work if it is not absorbed by your stomach or small intestine due to excess acid in your gut.

5. Many drugs will not work unless the drug is converted into a new medication in your liver. You may have a genetic mutation which prevents this conversion.

6. Your dose of medication may not be sufficient.

7. Your medicine may not be potent enough.

8. Most drugs need to be absorbed from your stomach or small intestine to enter your blood stream. Abdominal surgery may not leave a way for a drug to get into your blood stream.

9. Your liver may filter a large portion of the drug before it gets to the proper receptor.

10. Your kidneys may excrete your drug too quickly before it has time to give you relief.

11. Some foods that you eat may interact with your medication causing your medication not to work.

12. Smoking may inhibit the effects of some medications.

13. Many medications are divided into subclasses. A change from one subclass to another subclass may be effective for your condition.

14. Other factors can affect how quickly a drug is absorbed. For example, most absorption of oral drugs occurs in the small intestine. If a patient has had large sections of the small intestine surgically removed, drug absorption decreases. If your body does not absorb enough drug, it may not work.

15. Pain and stress can also decrease the amount of drug absorbed by your body.

16. Drug tolerance occurs when a patient develops a decreased response to a drug over time. You then require a larger dose of medication to produce the same response.

17. Some generic drugs may not work as well as the brand name drugs.

18. Your gender may affect how your drug works.

19. Medications may be given by mouth, by patch, by suppository, by injection or by nasal spray. If one form of drug is ineffective another form may work.

20. Some drugs compete for the same receptor (e.g. Narcan and Morphine where Narcan pushes the Morphine off the mu receptor which stops the effects of the Morphine).

21. You must read all the instructions and warnings that come with your medication for your drug to work effectively.

If your sleep medications do not work, you may have sleep apnea. Sleep apnea is a serious condition that leads not only to daytime sleepiness but also to depression and health problems. Sleep apnea is diagnosed with a sleep study, and treated with continuous positive airway pressure (CPAP) a mask worn over the mouth and nose at night that keeps the air moving continuously so the airway can't collapse. Some of the symptoms associated with sleep apnea include snoring loudly, excessive sleepiness during the day, insomnia, difficulty in concentrating, dry throat, and headaches in the morning and general body weakness or fatigue during the day. Gender, smoking, old age, heart disorders, weight and race are all factors that may determine the chances of an individual developing sleep apnea.

Sleep apnea is a condition in which the affected individual is constantly interrupted from sleep due to irregular breathing patterns. Sleep apnea is a condition that causes a person's sleep to be interrupted due to the brain's failure to communicate. When a person's sleep is interrupted due to relaxation of throat muscles, the condition is called obstructive sleep apnea.

Common symptoms of sleep apnea include hypersomnia, heavy snoring, a temporary inability to breathe, and abrupt awakenings short of breath, morning headaches, and attention problems. There are two primary types of sleep apnea: obstructive sleep apnea and central sleep apnea. Cheyne-stokes respiration, another name for central sleep apnea, is a neurological variant of sleep apnea. The respiratory system cycles between apnea and hyperapnea, or fast breathing. Clinical research has shown that not only are sleeping pills less effective than behavioral treatment for the treatment of chronic insomnia, but sleeping pills often make insomnia worse. The problem with pills include memory problems, morning drowsiness, changes in appetite, headaches, heartburn, shaking, stomach upset, and changes in testosterone and the menstrual cycle.

Anti-arrhythmic drugs used to treat heart rhythm problems can cause insomnia and other sleep difficulties. Beta blockers, used for high blood pressure, arrhythmias, and angina, increase the chance of insomnia, awakenings at night, and nightmares. Additionally, some cholesterol-lowering drugs have been linked to poor sleep. Theophylline, an asthma medication that is sometimes used to ease inflammation and help clear airways, can cause insomnia, as well as daytime jitters. Corticosteroids, such as prednisone, are frequently prescribed for asthma and can cause similar medication side effects. About 20 percent of people who take antidepressants known as selective serotonin reuptake inhibitors, (SSRIs), such as fluoxetine (Prozac), sertraline (Zoloft), and paroxetine (Paxil), experience sleep problems.

Nicotine patches used to help people quit smoking work by delivering small doses of nicotine into the bloodstream, and one common medication side effect is insomnia. Attention-deficit hyperactivity disorder is usually treated with stimulant-like medicines that boost alertness, but can lead to insomnia.

An underactive thyroid gland can cause extreme sleepiness during the day, but some drugs used to treat the condition can result in insomnia. Decongestants can cause insomnia. Some people taking St. John's wort for depression have reported overstimulation and insomnia. The most common side effect of all types of statins is muscle pain, which can keep people who take them awake at night and unable to rest. Sleeping pills can stop working as your body develops a tolerance to the medication.

Be aware that sleep medications only add about 20 to 40 minutes of sleep to your night. The side effects of sleep medications such as delayed reaction time, dizziness and memory problems, can be serious. Remember that alcohol becomes a stimulant about three to four hours after you drink it and can cause insomnia. If you don't have apnea, some physicians recommend cognitive behavioral therapy instead of medications.

## 30. Laxatives

Constipation is a symptom, not a disease. Constipation is a condition in which a person has difficulty in eliminating solid waste from the body, and the feces are hard and dry. Constipation can occur when a person's digestive system, for one reason or another, does not function properly. Different classifications of pathophysiological subgroups exist; the most common one is as follows: functional constipation, irritable bowel syndrome (IBS) or outlet obstruction. Constipation-promoting factors include chronic illnesses, immobility, neurologic and psychiatric conditions, and medicines used like morphine.

Constipation is commonly understood as having infrequent or difficult bowel movements, as well as having fewer than three bowel movements per week. Each person can experience constipation differently. While constipation symptoms are not the same for everyone, there tend to be some common signs and symptoms: Painful, difficult bowel movements, dry, hard stools, excessive straining, abdominal discomfort, and fewer than three bowel movements per week.

Constipation can be caused by certain diet and lifestyle choices, as well as physiological changes and certain medications. Sometimes it is not always easy to anticipate what will cause constipation; and it is not always predictable. Below is a list of the more common constipation causes. Diets with high fat and refined sugar, low fiber, dehydration, inactivity, lack of exercise, pregnancy, aging, antacids, calcium supplements and opiates may cause constipation.

Laxatives stimulate defecation and include: hyperosmolar drugs, dietary fiber and related bulk-forming substances, emollients, stimulants and lubricants.

There are different types of medications to treat constipation: bowel oral stimulant tablets which stimulate the muscles in your bowel to expel feces. This medication takes overnight to work.

Stimulant suppositories work in the same manner but work almost immediately. These drugs soften the stool in the intestine, making it easier to pass the feces. A stool softener works gradually. Osmotic drugs draw water into the bowel, providing softer stools and increases frequency of bowel movements and work in 1-3 days. A bulk forming laxative absorbs more fluid in the intestines, making the stool bigger, giving you the urge to pass the feces. This drug takes 1-2 days to work. Lubricant laxatives are another class of laxative, which coats the wall of the intestine so that stools can pass through more easily. A lubricant laxative works in 6 to 8 hours.

Treatment should be graded and should start with lifestyle and diet changes. Any medication that can cause constipation should be stopped if possible. Further steps include the use of bulk-forming agents, osmotic laxatives. The use of bulk-forming agents, osmotic laxatives should be used for treatment initially. Fiber and bulk laxatives decrease abdominal pain and improve stool consistency.

Bulk laxatives include: psyllium, polycarbophil and methylcellulose. Lubricating agents include mineral oil. Stimulant laxatives include surface-acting agents, docusate, bile acids, diphenyl methane derivatives, phenolphthalein, bisacodyl, sodium picosulfate, ricinoleic acid, castor oil, anthraquinones, senna, cascara, sagrada and aloes.

Osmotic agents include magnesium and phosphate salts, lactulose, sorbitol, glycerin suppositories, and polyethylene glycol.

The elderly frequently require laxatives because of lack of mobility and polypharmacy. Treatment is the same as for younger adults, with an emphasis on changing lifestyle and diet. For immobility, it is better to use stimulant laxatives instead of bulking agents. Senna-fiber combinations are more effective than lactulose. It is important to try to stop potentially constipating drugs.

In pregnancy one should use dietary fiber and increased fluid intake. In diabetic patients, bulk-forming laxatives are safe and useful for those unable or unwilling to increase dietary fiber.

Diabetics should avoid stimulant laxatives such as lactulose and sorbitol, since their metabolites may influence blood-glucose levels, especially in patients with type 1 diabetes.

In general, medications may not work for the following reasons:

1. Most drugs are manufactured for a specific ailment. If your diagnosis is wrong, and if you were prescribed a specific drug for a disease, you will not receive any relief.

2. Your prescribed drug may be adversely affected by your hormones.

3. Other drugs that you are taking may interfere with your medicine. Drug-drug interactions occur when two or more drugs react with each other. Drug-food/beverage interactions result from drugs reacting with foods or beverages. Drug-condition interactions may occur when an existing medical condition makes certain drugs potentially harmful

4. Your drug won't work if it is not absorbed by your stomach or small intestine due to excess acid in your gut.

5. Many drugs will not work unless the drug is converted into a new medication in your liver. You may have a genetic mutation which prevents this conversion.

6. Your dose of medication may not be sufficient.

7. Your medicine may not be potent enough.

8. Most drugs need to be absorbed from your stomach or small intestine to enter your blood stream. Abdominal surgery may not leave a way for a drug to get into your blood stream.

9. Your liver may filter a large portion of the drug before it gets to the proper receptor.

10. Your kidneys may excrete your drug too quickly before it has time to give you relief.

11. Some foods that you eat may interact with your medication causing your medication not to work.

12. Smoking may inhibit the effects of some medications.

13. Many medications are divided into subclasses. A change from one subclass to another subclass may be effective for your condition.

14. Other factors can affect how quickly a drug is absorbed. For example, most absorption of oral drugs occurs in the small intestine. If a patient has had large sections of the small intestine surgically removed, drug absorption decreases. If your body does not absorb enough drug, it may not work.

15. Pain and stress can also decrease the amount of drug absorbed by your body.

16. Drug tolerance occurs when a patient develops a decreased response to a drug over time. You then require a larger dose of medication to produce the same response.

17. Some generic drugs may not work as well as the brand name drugs.

18. Your gender may affect how your drug works.

19. Medications may be given by mouth, by patch, by suppository, by injection or by nasal spray. If one form of drug is ineffective another form may work.

20. Some drugs compete for the same receptor (e.g. Narcan and Morphine where Narcan pushes the Morphine off the mu receptor which stops the effects of the Morphine).

21. You must read all the instructions and warnings that come with your medication for your drug to work effectively.

Constipation can arise from stress or poor eating habits. Laxatives don't work sometimes because they draw the fluid out of your bowel. There are four different types of products for preventing or treating constipation. If one class does not work, you should try another class of laxative.

1. Bulking agents with food such as bran or products such as Citrucel, Metamucil, Fibercon, or Perdiem ease constipation by absorbing more fluid in the intestines. This makes the stool bigger, and softer which allows you to pass the stool. Regular use of bulking agents is safe and often lets you have more frequent stools.

2. Stool softeners such as Colace lubricate and soften the stool in the intestine, making it easier to pass the stool. Stool

softeners do not often cause problems but they don't work as well if you don't drink sufficient amounts of water during the day.

3. Osmotic laxatives such as Fleet Phospho-Soda, Milk of Magnesia, or Miralax and nonabsorbable sugars such as lactulose or sorbitol hold fluids in the intestine and draw fluids into the intestine from other tissue and blood vessels. This extra fluid in the intestines makes the stool softer and easier to pass.

4. Stimulant laxatives such as Correctol, Dulcolax, Ex-Lax, Feen-a-Mint, or Senokot speed up how fast a stool moves through the intestines by irritating the lining of the intestines. Regular use of stimulant laxatives is not recommended. Stimulant laxatives change the tone and feeling in the large intestine and you can become dependent on using laxatives all the time to have a bowel movement.

Although laxatives have been around for a long time, there is a lack of high-quality evidence about exactly how effective they are and whether certain laxatives are better than others. Unless there is a reason why specific laxatives may be more suitable than others, most adults should try using a bulk-forming laxative first. These usually start to work after about two or three days. If your stools remain hard, try using an osmotic laxative in addition to, or instead of, a bulk-forming laxative. If your stools are soft, but you still find them difficult to pass, try taking a stimulant laxative in addition to a bulk-forming laxative.

Osmotic laxatives usually start to work after about 2 or 3 days, while stimulant laxatives usually have an effect within 6 to 12 hours. Some laxatives are also designed to be taken at certain parts of the day such as the first thing in the morning or last thing at night. Make sure you carefully read the patient information leaflet that comes with your medication, so you know how to take it properly. Do not get into the habit of taking laxatives every day to ease your constipation, because this can be harmful.

## 31. Autoimmune drugs

Immune system disorders cause abnormally low activity or over activity of the immune system. In cases of immune system over activity, the body attacks and damages its own tissues which are called autoimmune diseases. Immune deficiency diseases decrease the body's ability to fight invaders, causing vulnerability to infections. In response to an unknown trigger, the immune system may begin producing antibodies that instead of fighting infections, attack the body's own tissues. Treatment for autoimmune diseases generally focuses on reducing immune system activity. There are more than 80 different types of autoimmune disorders.

More common disorders include: Rheumatoid arthritis where the immune system produces antibodies that attach to the linings of your joints. Immune system cells then attack the joints, causing inflammation. People with Systemic lupus erythematosus develop autoimmune antibodies that can attach to tissues throughout the body. The joints, lungs, blood cells, nerves, and kidneys are affected in lupus. Inflammatory bowel disease (IBD attacks the lining of the intestines. Ulcerative colitis and Crohn's disease are the two major forms of IBD. In Multiple sclerosis the immune system attacks nerve cells, causing pain, blindness, weakness, poor coordination, and muscle spasms. In Type 1 diabetes mellitus antibodies attack and destroy insulin producing cells in the pancreas. In the Guillain-Barre syndrome the immune system attacks the nerves controlling muscles in the legs. In psoriasis, overactive immune system cells collect in the skin, producing silvery, scaly lesions on the skin. In Graves' disease, the immune system produces antibodies that stimulate the thyroid gland to release excess amounts of thyroid hormone. In Hasimoto's disease antibodies produced by the immune system attack the thyroid gland and cause low levels. In Myasthenia gravis antibodies bind to nerves and make them unable to stimulate muscles. In Vasculitis the immune system attacks and damages blood vessels.

Normally the immune system's white blood cells help protect your body from harmful substances, called antigens. Examples of antigens include bacteria, viruses, toxins, cancer cells, and blood or tissues from another person or species. The immune system produces antibodies that destroy these harmful substances. In patients with an autoimmune disorder, the immune system can't tell the difference between healthy body tissue and antigens. The result is an immune response that destroys normal body tissues. This response is a hypersensitivity reaction similar to the response in allergic conditions. In allergies, the immune system reacts to an outside substance that it normally would ignore. With autoimmune disorders, the immune system reacts to normal body tissues that it would normally ignore.

The mechanism that causes tour immune system to no longer tell the difference between healthy body tissues and antigens is unknown. An autoimmune disorder may result in destruction of one or more types of body tissue or an abnormal growth of an organ. An autoimmune disorder may affect one or more organ or tissue types. A person may have more than one autoimmune disorder at the same time. Although there are many different types of autoimmune diseases and they can affect many different organs, they are all similar in that they are an immune response caused by systemic inflammation that causes your body to attack itself. If your immune system deems any foreign substance dangerous, your body will normally produce antibodies to ward off these substances.

There are many underlying factors that can cause people to develop an autoimmune condition. There is an underlying genetic component. However, whether these genes get expressed or turned on is caused by many factors, such as toxins from heavy metals like mercury or mycotoxins from molds, infections and gluten intolerance. If you suspect that you have an autoimmune disease, it important for your doctor to identify and treat the underlying cause. Your doctor may prescribe medications such as anti-inflammatory drugs, steroids, or immunosuppressants. Treatments involving immunosuppressant drugs can increase the risk of severe infections and cancer when taken for long periods of time.

Treatment for autoimmune diseases generally focuses on reducing immune system activity. Treatments for rheumatoid arthritis can include various oral or injectable medications that reduce your immune system over activity.

People with Systemic lupus erythematosus often require daily oral prednisone, a steroid that reduces immune system function. The goals of treatment are to: reduce symptoms, control the autoimmune process and maintain the body's ability to fight disease. When finding the right treatment for your autoimmune the goals of treatment are to relieve symptoms, preserve organ function, and target disease mechanisms.

The choice of autoimmune disease treatment will depend on the type of disease, how severe the disease is, and the symptoms of the disease. Generally, treatment options have one of three goals: relieving symptoms, preserving organ function and targeting disease mechanisms.

The interferon drugs are considered to be safe. Most of the side effects that do occur stem from the injection itself, including redness, warmth, itching, or dimpling of the skin over the injection site. With the interferon drugs, it's common to have flu-like symptoms: aches, fatigue, fever, and chills, but these should fade within a few months. The interferon drugs can also slightly increase your risk for real infections by lowering the number of white blood cells that help your immune system fight off illnesses.

Relieving symptoms may involve medication or surgery. When an autoimmune disease threatens organs, autoimmune disease treatment may be needed to prevent damage. Such treatments may include drugs to control an inflamed kidney in people with lupus, or insulin injections that can regulate blood sugar in people with diabetes. Although these treatments will not stop the autoimmune disease, they can save organ function and help people live with disease-related complications. Some drugs may also be used to target how the disease works. In other words, they can suppress the immune system. Autoimmune disorder medications include cyclophosphamide (Cytoxan, etanercept (Enbrel). Autoimmune diseases include ankylosing spondylitis, juvenile rheumatoid arthritis, psoriasis, psoriatic arthritis and rheumatoid arthritis

Methotrexate It is used as a treatment for some autoimmune diseases, including rheumatoid arthritis, juvenile dermatomyositis, psoriasis, psoriatic arthritis, lupus, sarcoidosis, Crohn's disease, eczema and many forms of vasculitis. Methotrexate is an antimetabolite and antifolate drug. It is used in treatment of cancer as well.

In general, your medications may not work for the following reasons:

1. Most drugs are manufactured for a specific ailment. If your diagnosis is wrong, and if you were prescribed a specific drug for a disease, you will not receive any relief.

2. Your prescribed drug may be adversely affected by your hormones.

3. Other drugs that you are taking may interfere with your medicine. Drug-drug interactions occur when two or more drugs react with each other. Drug-food/beverage interactions result from drugs reacting with foods or beverages. Drug-condition interactions may occur when an existing medical condition makes certain drugs potentially harmful.

4. Your drug won't work if it is not absorbed by your stomach or small intestine due to excess acid in your gut.

5. Many drugs will not work unless the drug is converted into a new medication in your liver. You may have a genetic mutation which prevents this conversion.

6. Your dose of medication may not be sufficient.

7. Your medicine may not be potent enough.

8. Most drugs need to be absorbed from your stomach or small intestine to enter your blood stream. Abdominal surgery may not leave a way for a drug to get into your blood stream.

9. Your liver may filter a large portion of the drug before it gets to the proper receptor.

10. Your kidneys may excrete your drug too quickly before it has time to give you relief.

11. Some foods that you eat may interact with your medication causing your medication not to work.

12. Smoking may inhibit the effects of some medications.

13. Many medications are divided into subclasses. A change from one subclass to another subclass may be effective for your condition.

14. Other factors can affect how quickly a drug is absorbed. For example, most absorption of oral drugs occurs in the small intestine. If a patient has had large sections of the small intestine surgically removed, drug absorption decreases. If your body does not absorb enough drug, it may not work.

15. Pain and stress can also decrease the amount of drug absorbed by your body.

16. Drug tolerance occurs when a patient develops a decreased response to a drug over time. You then require a larger dose of medication to produce the same response.

17. Some generic drugs may not work as well as the brand name drugs.

18. Your gender may affect how your drug works.

19. Medications may be given by mouth, by patch, by suppository, by injection or by nasal spray. If one form of drug is ineffective another form may work.

20. Some drugs compete for the same receptor (e.g. Narcan and Morphine where Narcan pushes the Morphine off the mu receptor which stops the effects of the Morphine).

21. You must read all the instructions and warnings that come with your medication for your drug to work effectively.

## 32. Birth Control Pills

Oral contraceptives (birth control pills) are medications that prevent pregnancy. Pregnancy is the physical condition of a woman carrying an unborn offspring inside her body, from fertilization to birth. Oral contraceptives are one method of birth control. Oral contraceptives are hormonal preparations that may contain combinations of the hormones estrogen and progestin or progestin alone.

Combinations of estrogen and progestin prevent pregnancy by inhibiting the release of the hormones luteinizing hormone (LH) and follicle stimulating hormone (FSH) from the pituitary gland in the brain. LH and FSH play key roles for the development of the egg and preparation of the lining of the uterus for implantation of the embryo. Progestin also makes the uterine mucus that surrounds the egg more difficult for sperm to penetrate and; therefore, for fertilization to take place. In some women, progestin inhibits ovulation.

Birth control pills contain hormones that suppress ovulation. During ovulation an egg is released from the ovaries. Without ovulation, there is no egg to be fertilized and pregnancy cannot occur. There are 2 types of birth control pills: the combined pill and the minipill. The combined pill contains both estrogen and progestin, while the minipill contains only progestin.

The progestin in the minipill may prevent ovulation; however, it may not do this reliably each month. The minipill works further by thickening the mucous around the cervix and preventing sperm from entering the uterus. The lining of the uterus is also affected in a way that prevents fertilized eggs from implanting into the wall of the uterus.

The minipill is taken every day. You may not have a period while taking the minipill. If you do have periods that means you are still ovulating, and your risk for pregnancy is greater.

Combination birth control pills come in either 21 or 28-day packs. You take one pill each day at the same time for 21 days. If you have a 21-day pack, you stop taking birth control pills for 7 days at the end of the pack. If you are taking a 28-day pack, you continue taking pills every day.

There are different types of combination birth control pills that contain estrogen and progestin that are referred to as "monophasic," "biphasic," or "triphasic." Monophasic birth control pills deliver the same amount of estrogen and progestin every day. Biphasic birth control pills deliver the same amount of estrogen every day for the first 21 days of the cycle. During the first half of the cycle, the progestin/estrogen ratio is lower to allow the lining of the uterus (endometrium) to thicken as it normally does during the menstrual cycle. During the second half of the cycle, the progestin/estrogen ratio is higher to allow the normal shedding of the lining of the uterus to occur. Triphasic birth control pills have constant or changing estrogen concentrations and varying progestin concentrations throughout the cycle. There is no evidence that bi or triphasic oral contraceptives are safer or superior to monophasic oral contraceptives in their effectiveness for the prevention of pregnancy.

Women just starting to take birth control pills should use additional contraception for the first seven days of use because pregnancy may occur during this period. If women forget to take the pills, pregnancy may result. If a single tablet is forgotten, it should be taken as soon as it is realized that it is forgotten.

In general, your medications may not work for the following reasons:

1. Most drugs are manufactured for a specific ailment. If your diagnosis is wrong, and if you were prescribed a specific drug for a disease, you will not receive any relief.

2. Your prescribed drug may be adversely affected by your hormones.

3. Other drugs that you are taking may interfere with your medicine. Drug-drug interactions occur when two or more drugs react with each other. Drug-food/beverage interactions result from drugs reacting with foods or beverages. Drug-

condition interactions may occur when an existing medical condition makes certain drugs potentially harmful.

    4. Your drug won't work if it is not absorbed by your stomach or small intestine due to excess acid in your gut.

    5. Many drugs will not work unless the drug is converted into a new medication in your liver. You may have a genetic mutation which prevents this conversion.

    6. Your dose of medication may not be sufficient.

    7. Your medicine may not be potent enough.

    8. Most drugs need to be absorbed from your stomach or small intestine to enter your blood stream. Abdominal surgery may not leave a way for a drug to get into your blood stream.

    9. Your liver may filter a large portion of the drug before it gets to the proper receptor.

    10. Your kidneys may excrete your drug too quickly before it has time to give you relief.

    11. Some foods that you eat may interact with your medication causing your medication not to work.

    12. Smoking may inhibit the effects of some medications.

    13. Many medications are divided into subclasses. A change from one subclass to another subclass may be effective for your condition.

14. Other factors can affect how quickly a drug is absorbed. For example, most absorption of oral drugs occurs in the small intestine. If a patient has had large sections of the small intestine surgically removed, drug absorption decreases. If your body does not absorb enough drug, it may not work.

15. Pain and stress can also decrease the amount of drug absorbed by your body.

16. Drug tolerance occurs when a patient develops a decreased response to a drug over time. You then require a larger dose of medication to produce the same response.

17. Some generic drugs may not work as well as the brand name drugs.

18. Your gender may affect how your drug works.

19. Medications may be given by mouth, by patch, by suppository, by injection or by nasal spray. If one form of drug is ineffective another form may work.

20. Some drugs compete for the same receptor (e.g. Narcan and Morphine where Narcan pushes the Morphine off the mu receptor which stops the effects of the Morphine).

21. You must read all the instructions and warnings that come with your medication for your drug to work effectively.

A number of medications, including some antibiotics and anti-seizure medications, can decrease the blood levels of oral contraceptive hormones and make the birth control pills less effective. Keep in mind, even the most effective birth control methods can fail. But your chances of getting pregnant are lowest if the method you choose always is used correctly and every time you have sex.

Antibiotics taken by mouth can potentially decrease the effectiveness of birth control pills (the estrogen containing oral contraceptives). This occurs because, in addition to killing the bacteria responsible for causing the current illness or infection, oral antibiotics also kill the normal bacteria that live in the stomach that are responsible for activating the birth control pill. As a result, the oral contraceptive may be less effective.

## 33. Cardiac Drugs

The heart, arteries, veins, and lymphatics make up the cardiovascular system. There are several classes of drugs used to treat cardiovascular disorders. They include: inotropic, antiarrhythmic, antihypertensive drugs in heart failure, antianginal, and antilipemic medications. Antihypertensive medications were mentioned in a previous chapter.

Inotropic drugs increase the force of the heart's contractions. Some cardiac glycosides also slow the heart rate. Inotropic drugs work by having an effect on the force of cardiac muscular contraction. Digoxin is an inotropic drug which means that it has an effect on the force of the heart muscular contraction. This means that it helps a weakened heart work more efficiently to send blood through your body. It strengthens the force of the heart muscle's contractions and may improve circulation. It is a prescription drug used to help treat irregular heartbeat and improve symptoms of fatigue caused by heart failure. Elderly people taking higher doses of digoxin may become delirious or confused and feel weak or tired. Antacids, barbiturates, cholestyramine resin, kaolin and pectin, neomycin, metoclopramide, rifampin, and sulfasalazine reduce the therapeutic effects of digoxin.

Vasodilators are used to treat heart failure and control high blood pressure by relaxing the blood vessels so blood can flow more easily through your body. Vasodilators are medications that open blood vessels. They work directly on the muscles in the walls of your arteries, preventing the muscles from tightening and the walls from narrowing. As a result, blood flows more easily through your arteries, your heart doesn't have to pump as hard and your blood pressure is reduced. In essence, a vasodilator is an agent that widens the blood vessels, which in turn decreases resistance to blood flow and lowers your blood pressure. Arterial dilator drugs are commonly used to treat systemic and pulmonary hypertension, heart failure and angina. They reduce arterial pressure by decreasing systemic vascular resistance. Venous dilators reduce venous pressure, which reduces preload on the heart thereby decreasing cardiac output. Most vasodilators act on both arteries and veins, and therefore are termed mixed or balanced dilators. Some drugs primarily dilate resistance vessels (arterial dilators; e.g., hydralazine), while others primarily affect venous capacitance vessels (venous dilators; e.g., nitroglycerine).

ACE inhibitors are a type of medication that widens arteries to lower blood pressure and make it easier for the heart to pump blood. This class of drugs is used primarily for the treatment of hypertension and congestive heart failure. In treating heart disease, ACE inhibitors are usually used with other medications. ACE inhibitors are typically used when beta-adrenergic blockers or diuretics are ineffective.

Commonly prescribed ACE inhibitors include: benazepril, captopril, enalapril, enalaprilat, fosinopril, Lisinopril, moexipril, quinapril, Ramipril and trandolapril. ACE inhibitors can cause headaches, dizziness, fatigue, nausea, dry cough, angioedema that is a swelling of the face, tongue and throat and impaired kidney function. ACE inhibitors work to relax blood vessels by blocking the production of an enzyme in your body called angiotensin II.

Angiotensin II Receptor Blocker (ARBs): ARBs are used to decrease blood pressure in people with heart failure. ARBs decrease certain chemicals that narrow the blood vessels so blood can flow more easily through your body. Angiotensin II receptor blockers (ARBs) lower blood pressure by blocking the vasoconstrictive effects of angiotensin II. Specific drugs include: candesartan cilexetil, eprosartan, irbesartan, losartan, olmesartan, telmisartan and valsartan. blood vessels enlarge (dilate) and blood pressure is reduced. Reduced blood pressure makes it easier for the heart to pump blood and can improve heart failure.

Beta-blockers block the effects of adrenaline and improve the heart's ability to perform. Beta-adrenergic blockers, the most widely used adrenergic blockers; prevent stimulation of the sympathetic nervous system by inhibiting the action of catecholamines at beta-adrenergic receptors. Beta-adrenergic blockers can be selective or nonselective. Non-selective beta-adrenergic blockers affect: beta1 receptor sites (located mainly in the heart), beta2 receptor sites (located in the bronchi, blood vessels, and uterus).

Nonselective beta-adrenergic blockers include carteolol, carvedilol, labetalol, levobunolol, metipranolol, penbutolol, pindolol, sotalol, nadolol, propranolol, and timolol. include acebutolol, atenolol, betaxolol, bisoprolol, esmolol, and metoprolol. Selective Beta blockers include carteolol, carvedilol, labetalol, levobunolol, metipranolol, penbutolol, pindolol, sotalol, nadolol, propranolol, and timolol. Decreased effects can occur when rifampin, antacids, calcium salts, barbiturates, or anti-inflammatories, such as indomethacin and salicylates, are taken with beta-adrenergic blockers. Beta-blockers have been shown to prevent myocardial infarctions as well.

Calcium channel blockers are used to treat hypertension, angina and arrhythmias. Calcium channel blockers affect the movement of calcium in the cells of the heart and blood vessels. As a result, the drugs relax blood vessels. Calcium channel blockers are commonly used to prevent angina that doesn't respond to other angina medications and include: amlodipine, diltiazem, nicardipine, nifedipine, and verapamil.

Calcium channel blockers, or calcium antagonists, treat a variety of conditions, such as high blood pressure as well. Some calcium channel blockers have the added benefit of slowing your heart rate, which can further reduce blood pressure, relieve chest pain and control irregular heartbeats. Examples of calcium channel blockers include: Amlodipine (Norvasc), Diltiazem (Cardizem, Tiazac), Felodipine, Isradipine, Nicardipine (Cardene SR), Nifedipine (Procardia), Nisoldipine (Sular) and Verapamil (Calan, Verelan, Covera-HS).

In some cases, your doctor might prescribe a calcium channel blocker along with other high blood pressure medications. Calcium channel blockers may not be as effective as diuretics, beta blockers or angiotensin-converting enzyme (ACE) inhibitors at lowering blood pressure. Because of this, calcium channel blockers aren't usually the first medication you'd be prescribed to lower your blood pressure. Calcium channel blockers interact with grapefruit products as well.

Be aware that a benign parathyroid tumor can cause uncontrolled hypertension in about 10%-15% of patients. Parathyroid tumor(s) usually are diagnosed from a high blood calcium level. However, new studies demonstrate that some patients do NOT have a high calcium level but do have a parathyroid tumor. If you have uncontrolled hypertension, a parathyroid tumor should be ruled out. High blood pressure can become difficult to control over time resulting in need for more medication. It is not uncommon to be prescribed 3-4 medications to control high blood pressure.

However, many factors may play a role in blood pressure control. A diet low in salt and adherence to medication regimen prescribed by your doctor is very important in controlling blood pressure. Unhealthy lifestyle practices may play a major role in uncontrolled high blood pressure. Smoking, obesity, high cholesterol, and lack of exercise may contribute to uncontrolled blood pressure. Usually, it's not just one single issue but factors that contribute to the problem. Other drugs can interfere with blood pressure control, including pain relievers (NSAIDs), oral contraceptives and nasal decongestants.

Antianginal drugs treat angina by reducing myocardial oxygen demand (reducing the amount of oxygen the heart needs to do its work), by increasing the supply of oxygen to the heart, or both. Anti-angina drugs include nitrates for the treatment of acute angina and beta-adrenergic blockers for the long-term prevention of angina. Nitrates are used for the treatment of acute angina while beta-adrenergic blockers are used for the long-term prevention of angina. This class of drug includes amyl nitrite, isosorbide dinitrate, isosorbide mononitrate and nitroglycerin. calcium channel blockers (used when other drugs fail to prevent angina). Nitrates cause the smooth muscle of the veins and, to a lesser extent, the arteries to relax and dilate. Absorption of sublingual nitrates may be delayed when taken with an anticholinergic drug.

Anti lipidemic drugs are used as adjunct therapy with diet therapy to prevent a heart attack and the drug choice is based on the lipid profile of the patient. This class of drug reduces serum lipid levels. Antilipemic drugs are used to lower abnormally high blood levels of lipids, such as cholesterol, triglycerides, and phospholipids. Your cholesterol levels are an important measure of heart health. With respect to high-density lipoprotein (HDL) cholesterol, the higher the better. Too much low-density lipoprotein (LDL), cholesterol is a serious problem that can lead to heart disease. LDL cholesterol is the main source of cholesterol buildup and blockage in the arteries. On the other hand, high-density lipoprotein (HDL), cholesterol helps prevent cholesterol from building up in the arteries. The risk of developing coronary artery disease increases when serum lipid levels are elevated. The therapeutic effects of antilipemic drugs include decreased cholesterol and decreased triglycerides. The classes of antilipemic drugs include: bile-sequestering drugs, fibric acid derivatives, 3-hydroxy-3-methylglutaryl coenzyme A reductase inhibitors (statins), nicotinic acid and cholesterol absorption inhibitors.

Statins lower lipid levels by interfering with cholesterol synthesis. Taking a statin drug with amiodarone, clarithromycin, cyclosporine, erythromycin, fluconazole, gemfibrozil, itraconazole, ketoconazole, or niacin increases the risk of myopathy or rhabdomyolysis which is a potentially fatal breakdown of skeletal muscle.

Nicotinic acid is a water-soluble vitamin that decreases cholesterol, triglyceride, and apolipoprotein B-100 levels and increases the HDL level. Cholesterol absorption inhibitors inhibit the absorption of cholesterol and related phytosterols from the intestine. Ezetimibe is an example of a drug in this class.

Why won't my medication work?

In general, your medications may not work for the following reasons:

1. Most drugs are manufactured for a specific ailment. If your diagnosis is wrong, and if you were prescribed a specific drug for a disease, you will not receive any relief.

2. Your prescribed drug may be adversely affected by your hormones.

3. Other drugs that you are taking may interfere with your medicine. Drug-drug interactions occur when two or more drugs react with each other. Drug-food/beverage interactions result from drugs reacting with foods or beverages. Drug-

condition interactions may occur when an existing medical condition makes certain drugs potentially harmful.

4. Your drug won't work if it is not absorbed by your stomach or small intestine due to excess acid in your gut.

5. Many drugs will not work unless the drug is converted into a new medication in your liver. You may have a genetic mutation which prevents this conversion.

6. Your dose of medication may not be sufficient.

7. Your medicine may not be potent enough.

8. Most drugs need to be absorbed from your stomach or small intestine to enter your blood stream. Abdominal surgery may not leave a way for a drug to get into your blood stream.

9. Your liver may filter a large portion of the drug before it gets to the proper receptor.

10. Your kidneys may excrete your drug too quickly before it has time to give you relief.

11. Some foods that you eat may interact with your medication causing your medication not to work.

12. Smoking may inhibit the effects of some medications.

13. Many medications are divided into subclasses. A change from one subclass to another subclass may be effective for your condition.

14. Other factors can affect how quickly a drug is absorbed. For example, most absorption of oral drugs occurs in the small intestine. If a patient has had large sections of the small intestine surgically removed, drug absorption decreases. If your body does not absorb enough drug, it may not work.

15. Pain and stress can also decrease the amount of drug absorbed by your body.

16. Drug tolerance occurs when a patient develops a decreased response to a drug over time. You then require a larger dose of medication to produce the same response.

17. Some generic drugs may not work as well as the brand name drugs.

18. Your gender may affect how your drug works.

19. Medications may be given by mouth, by patch, by suppository, by injection or by nasal spray. If one form of drug is ineffective, another form may work.

20. Some drugs compete for the same receptor (e.g. Narcan and Morphine where Narcan pushes the Morphine off the mu receptor which stops the effects of the Morphine).

21. You must read all the instructions and warnings that come with your medication for your drug to work effectively.

Drug interactions may interfere with the drugs described in this chapter. Grapefruit juice can lessen digoxin's ability to work. NSAIDs reduce the antihypertensive effects of ARBs.

Decreased beta blocker effects can occur when rifampin, antacids, calcium salts, barbiturates, or anti-inflammatories, such as indomethacin and salicylates are taken in patients using beta blockers. Verapamil and diltiazem increase the risk of digoxin toxicity, enhance the action of carbamazepine, and may cause myocardial depression. Absorption of sublingual nitrates may be delayed when taken with an anticholinergic drug which will make the nitrate slow to work. Bile-sequestering antilipemic drugs may bind with acidic drugs in the GI tract, decreasing their absorption and effectiveness. Fibric acid antilipemic drugs may bind with acidic drugs in the GI tract, decreasing their absorption and effectiveness. Lovastatin, rosuvastatin and simvastatin may increase the risk of bleeding when administered with warfarin. Bile-sequestering drugs (cholestyramine, colesevelam, and colestipol) can bind with nicotinic acid and decrease its effectiveness.

## 34. Pulmonary Drugs

There are different classes of drugs used to treat respiratory disorders. Drugs used to improve respiratory symptoms are available in inhalation and systemic formulations. These drugs include: beta2-adrenergic agonists, anticholinergics, corticosteroids and leukotriene modifiers. Beta2-adrenergic agonists are used to treat symptoms associated with asthma and chronic obstructive pulmonary disease

Bronchodilators are a type of medications that helps open the airways to make breathing easier. Broncho dilators are used to treat respiratory symptoms associated with asthma and chronic obstructive pulmonary disease. Albuterol, levalbuterol, and ipratropium are all short-acting bronchodilators. They come in the form of an inhaler or as a liquid that you can add to a nebulizer to inhale. Interactions are uncommon when using the inhaled forms.

Corticosteroids are a type of medication that reduces inflammation in the body, making air flow easier to the lungs. Corticosteroids are anti-inflammatory drugs available in inhaled and systemic forms for the short- and long-term control of asthma symptoms.

Leukotriene modifiers are used for the prevention and long-term control of mild asthma. Leukotriene receptor antagonists include: montelukast and zafirlukast. Leukotriene formation inhibitors include: zileuton. Zileuton is contraindicated in a patient with active liver disease.

Some doctors will prescribe theophylline when other treatments do not work, and theophylline works as an anti-inflammatory and relaxes the muscles in the airway and may be taken along with a bronchodilator. Xanthines, are also used to treat respiratory disorders. Theophylline and its salts are used as second- or third-line therapy for the long-term control and prevention of symptoms related to: asthma, chronic bronchitis and emphysema.

Expectorants are used to thin mucus so it's cleared more easily out of the airways to help you breathe better. The most commonly used expectorant is guaifenesin. Expectorants reduce the thickness, adhesiveness, and surface tension of mucus, making it easier to clear from the airways. Guaifenesin is used to relieve symptoms due to bronchial asthma and bronchitis.

Antitussive drugs suppress coughing symptoms. The major antitussives include: benzonatate, codeine, dextromethorphan and hydrocodone bitartrate.

In general, medications may not work for the following reasons:

1. Most drugs are manufactured for a specific ailment. If your diagnosis is wrong, and if you were prescribed a specific drug for a disease, you will not receive any relief.

2. Your prescribed drug may be adversely affected by your hormones.

3. Other drugs that you are taking may interfere with your medicine. Drug-drug interactions occur when two or more drugs react with each other. Drug-food/beverage interactions result from drugs reacting with foods or beverages. Drug-condition interactions may occur when an existing medical condition makes certain drugs potentially harmful

4. Your drug won't work if it is not absorbed by your stomach or small intestine due to excess acid in your gut.

5. Many drugs will not work unless the drug is converted into a new medication in your liver. You may have a genetic mutation which prevents this conversion.

6. Your dose of medication may not be sufficient.

7. Your medicine may not be potent enough.

8. Most drugs need to be absorbed from your stomach or small intestine to enter your blood stream. Abdominal surgery may not leave a way for a drug to get into your blood stream.

9. Your liver may filter a large portion of the drug before it gets to the proper receptor.

10. Your kidneys may excrete your drug too quickly before it has time to give you relief.

11. Some foods that you eat may interact with your medication causing your medication not to work.

12. Smoking may inhibit the effects of some medications.

13. Many medications are divided into subclasses. A change from one subclass to another subclass may be effective for your condition.

14. Other factors can affect how quickly a drug is absorbed. For example, most absorption of oral drugs occurs in the small intestine. If a patient has had large sections of the small intestine surgically removed, drug absorption decreases. If your body does not absorb enough drug, it may not work.

15. Pain and stress can also decrease the amount of drug absorbed by your body.

16. Drug tolerance occurs when a patient develops a decreased response to a drug over time. You then require a larger dose of medication to produce the same response.

17. Some generic drugs may not work as well as the brand name drugs.

18. Your gender may affect how your drug works.

WHY WON'T MY MECIDICATION WORK? 313

19. Medications may be given by mouth, by patch, by suppository, by injection or by nasal spray. If one form of drug is ineffective another form may work.

20. Some drugs compete for the same receptor (e.g. Narcan and Morphine where Narcan pushes the Morphine off the mu receptor which stops the effects of the Morphine).

21. You must read all the instructions and warnings that come with your medication for your drug to work effectively.

Some causes of the lack of your pulmonary medications include the following reasons. Beta-adrenergic blockers decrease the bronchodilation effects of beta2-adrenergic agonists. Barbiturates, cholestyramine, rifampin, and phenytoin may decrease the effectiveness of corticosteroids, resulting in the need to increase the steroid dosage. Carbamazepine, phenobarbital, phenytoin, rifampin and St. John's wort increase theophylline metabolism, thus decreasing its effectiveness. Beta-adrenergic blockers decrease the bronchodilation effects of beta2-adrenergic agonists. Barbiturates, cholestyramine, rifampin, and phenytoin may decrease the effectiveness of corticosteroids. Barbiturates, cholestyramine, rifampin, and phenytoin may decrease the effectiveness of corticosteroids.

Smoking cigarettes or marijuana increases theophylline elimination and decreases effectiveness. Carbamazepine, phenobarbital, phenytoin, rifampin, St. John's wort, and charbroiled meats increase theophylline metabolism, thus decreasing its serum level and possibly its effectiveness. Furthermore, thyroid hormones may reduce theophylline levels and in doing so, you may not have any relief of your symptoms.

## 35. Blood Thinners

Blood clots can lead to strokes, heart attacks or other serious health conditions. Anticoagulants are a class of drugs that work to prevent the clotting of blood. If you have heart or blood vessel disease, or if you have poor blood flow to your brain, your doctor may prescribe a blood thinner. Blood thinners reduce the risk of heart attack and stroke by reducing the formation of blood clots in your arteries and veins. You may also take a blood thinner if you have: an abnormal heart rhythm called atrial fibrillation, have had heart valve surgery or have congenital heart defects. Blood thinners don't actually thin your blood. They keep harmful clots from forming in your veins and stop them from getting bigger.

The formation of a normal blood clot depends on a series of chemical interactions. Platelets form a plug to stop bleeding. Proteins in your blood called clotting factors cause a rapid chain reaction. It ends with a dissolved substance in your blood turning into long strands of fibrin. These get tangled up with the platelets in the plug to create a net that traps even more platelets and cells. Some medications like aspirin keep blood clots from occurring by preventing platelets from adhering together. Other medications prevent the formation of fibrin.

More than 2 million people take blood thinners every day to keep them from developing dangerous blood clots. There are different types of blood thinners. The most common blood thinner is warfarin called Coumadin. It was initially introduced in 1948 as a pesticide against rats and mice.

Blood thinners stop blood coagulation. Blood coagulation means that your body forms a clot. Several proteins involved in coagulation are called vitamin-K-dependent coagulation factors. A series of plasma proteins converts an inactive precursor into an active enzyme leading to the formation of a fibrin clot. Clot formation is usually good as it helps you stop bleeding if you have an injury. A clot can be harmful however, if it blocks one of your arteries to your heart, brain etc. Other medicines can change the way your blood thinner works. Your blood thinner can also change how other medicines work. High amounts of vitamin K can work against warfarin. Warfarin, aspirin and Plavix are the most widely used medications for blocking clot formation.

Increasing or decreasing the International Normalized Ratio, or INR, which is a measure of how quickly blood clots. Vitamins such as Vitamin K can lower a patient's INR, increasing the risk of forming dangerous clots. Some herbal products such as green tea, ginseng, danshen, bromelains, fenugreek and garlic-based supplements also react with blood thinners.

Newer blood thinners include: Apixaban (Eliquis), Dabigatran (Pradaxa), and Rivaroxaban (Xarelto). And since they wear off faster than warfarin, bleeding problems may not be as serious when they happen. Furthermore, vitamin K doesn't interfere with how they work. You must remain on warfarin if you have kidney failure or if you have mechanical heart valves. The newer medications may not be safe for those situations.

Coumadin works by decreasing the amount of vitamin K available for use in the body, which in turn reduces the efficiency of blood clot formation by the body. This is why you should monitor your intake of foods that are rich in vitamin K. Some foods with high vitamin K content include spinach, lettuce, alfalfa sprouts, asparagus, broccoli, cauliflower, and cabbage.

Heparin is usually given in the hospital directly into a blood vessel. Lovenox, also called enoxaparin, is a form of heparin called fractionated heparin. Lovenox does not require monitoring of its blood levels and it can be injected intramuscularly.

Newer anticoagulants include Pradaxa, Xarelto and Eliquis. Pradaxa was approved by the FDA for the prevention of stroke and blood clots in people with atrial fibrillation. Xarelto was approved, to treat atrial fibrillation. It had been approved earlier to lower the risk of blood clots after hip and knee replacements and to treat deep vein thrombosis, (blood clots that occur usually in the lower leg and thigh) and pulmonary embolism where a blood clot from a vein travels to an artery in the lungs and blocks blood flow.

Xarelto works by blocking Factor X, an enzyme needed for blood clots to form. Xarelto can cause bleeding, which can be serious, and rarely may lead to death. This is because this medication is a blood thinner medicine that reduces blood clotting. Xarelto side effects include uncontrolled internal bleeding, pulmonary embolism, deep vein thrombosis, ischemic strokes, embolic strokes, and in most severe cases death. Eliquis (apixaban) was approved to lower the risk of stroke and blood clots in patients with atrial fibrillation. Aspirin and Plavix work differently from warfarin and the other three drugs mentioned in that they prevent platelets in the blood from clumping together.

Foods that have natural anticoagulant properties that cause blood thinning include ginger, garlic, aniseed and celery seed. These foods can cause significant bleeding in patients taking blood thinners. Foods that contain high levels of vitamin E are also natural blood thinners.

In about one in four patients, the blood's ability to clot remained essentially unchanged with some of the anticoagulants mentioned. Those patients apparently had had more severe heart attacks and were more likely to suffer from blood clots and heart attacks in spite of taking a blood thinner.

# WHY WON'T MY MECIDICATION WORK?

In general, your medications may not work for the following reasons:

1. Most drugs are manufactured for a specific ailment. If your diagnosis is wrong, and if you were prescribed a specific drug for a disease, you will not receive any relief.

2. Your prescribed drug may be adversely affected by your hormones.

3. Other drugs that you are taking may interfere with your medicine. Drug-drug interactions occur when two or more drugs react with each other. Drug-food/beverage interactions result from drugs reacting with foods or beverages. Drug-condition interactions may occur when an existing medical condition makes certain drugs potentially harmful.

4. Your drug won't work if it is not absorbed by your stomach or small intestine due to excess acid in your gut.

5. Many drugs will not work unless the drug is converted into a new medication in your liver. You may have a genetic mutation which prevents this conversion.

6. Your dose of medication may not be sufficient.

7. Your medicine may not be potent enough.

8. Most drugs need to be absorbed from your stomach or small intestine to enter your blood stream. Abdominal surgery may not leave a way for a drug to get into your blood stream.

9. Your liver may filter a large portion of the drug before it gets to the proper receptor.

10. Your kidneys may excrete your drug too quickly before it has time to give you relief.

11. Some foods that you eat may interact with your medication causing your medication not to work.

12. Smoking may inhibit the effects of some medications.

13. Many medications are divided into subclasses. A change from one subclass to another subclass may be effective for your condition.

14. Other factors can affect how quickly a drug is absorbed. For example, most absorption of oral drugs occurs in the small intestine. If a patient has had large sections of the small intestine surgically removed, drug absorption decreases. If your body does not absorb enough drug, it may not work.

15. Pain and stress can also decrease the amount of drug absorbed by your body.

16. Drug tolerance occurs when a patient develops a decreased response to a drug over time. You then require a larger dose of medication to produce the same response.

17. Some generic drugs may not work as well as the brand name drugs.

18. Your gender may affect how your drug works.

WHY WON'T MY MECIDICATION WORK? 321

19. Medications may be given by mouth, by patch, by suppository, by injection or by nasal spray. If one form of drug is ineffective another form may work.

20. Some drugs compete for the same receptor (e.g. Narcan and Morphine where Narcan pushes the Morphine off the mu receptor which stops the effects of the Morphine).

21. You must read all the instructions and warnings that come with your medication for your drug to work effectively.

Researchers examined the effects of Plavix on 60 patients who were treated with angioplasties and devices known as stents that keep the arteries open. In addition to aspirin treatment, the patients all got a high dose of 300 milligrams of Plavix after their angioplasties and then received smaller, 75-milligram doses for three months. To measure the blood's ability to clot, researchers turned to a test that gauges how well blood components known as platelets stick together. In about one in four patients on Plavix, the blood's ability to clot remained essentially unchanged. Those patients apparently had more severe heart attacks and were more likely to suffer from blood clots and heart attacks after their operations. Further study is ongoing to determine the reason for this finding. Blood thinners significantly decrease your risk of blood clotting, but will not decrease the risk to zero. Blood thinners may not be able to lessen the strong blood-clotting tendency of an underlying disease, such as cancer. Interactions with other medications, food and alcohol are common with warfarin.

Alcohol can interact with anticoagulants as well, and your intake should be limited. Strawberries, seaweed, tofu and soy protein, soybean oil, green onions and green tea may increase your risk of blood clotting as well. Liver is high in vitamin K. Ginger and turmeric may affect the way your blood and should be limited when you are taking anticoagulants.

# Index

, anticholinergics 309

Abilify 165

absorption 3

addiction 57

adjuvant analgesics 156

Adverse drug reactions 92

agonist 2

Agonistic opioids 123

AIDS 227

angiotensin receptor blockers 174

antacids 183

antagonist 2

Anti lipidemic drugs 303

antibiotics 217

Anticoagulants 315

antidepressants 161

anti-inflammatory drugs 103

Anti-seizure drugs 147

Antitussive drugs 310

antiviral medications 219

anxiolytics 161

autoimmune diseases 283

Barbiturates 166

beta-adrenergic blockers 300

blood-brain barrier 5

Bronchodilators 309

calcium channel blockers 174, 301

Cancer stem cells 215

Chemotherapy 203

coagulates 322

cocaine 137

Constipation 275

Controlled Substances 34

cytochrome P450 enzymes 98

development of drugs 31

DHEA 237

diuretics 180

dopamin 168

Drug distribution 4

drug interaction 15

Drug metabolism 11

drug schedule 35

duration of action 6

elderly 76

erectile dysfunction 245

essential hypertension 174

estrogen 240

Euphoria 125

first-pass effect 5

follicle-stimulating hormone 235

GABA 255

Gender differences 22

Generic drugs 29

GERD 184

gouty arthritis 111

H-2 receptor blockers 185

Helicobacter pylori 183

herb 47

high-density lipoprotein 303

hormone 235

Hydromorphone 128

hypertension 173

Hypertension 173

Hypothyroidism 199

immune system. 283

Inotropic drugs 297

insomnia 265

in-teraction 13

intraurethral prostaglandin 251

isoenzymes 12

Laxatives 276

leukotriene modifiers 309

Lithium 166

low-density lipoprotein 303

Luteinizing hormone 235

marijuana 49

medication 1

Meperidine 128

minipill 292

Misoprostol 184

muscle relaxants 253, 254

NERD 190

neuropathic pain 147

Nicotine 169

Nitrates 302

norepinephrine 168

Novocain 135

NSAIDs 103

opioids 122

Oral contraceptives 291

overdose 14

Pharmacodynamics 1

Pharmacogenetic testing 102

Pharmacogenetics 95

Physical dependence 63

poor metabolizer 96

post-surgery pain 150

progesterone 241

proton pump inhibitors 184

psychoactive drug 159

Rectal administration 3

regional anesthesia 135

resistant hypertension 179

secondary hypertension 174

serotonin 168

SSRIs. 166

Tapentadol 129

testosterone 239

THC 49

thyroid medication 199

thyroid-stimulating hormone 235

Tolerance 63

Tramadol 127

Transdermal 3

type 2 diabetes 192

Uricosurics 110

## About the Author

William E. Ackerman III, M.D., is a fellowship trained, American Board of Anesthesiology certified anesthesiologist with American Board of Anesthesiology certification in Pain Medicine as well. He is in private practice and is the Medical Director and President of a Pain Medicine practice. Dr. Ackerman has had an extensive academic career. Dr. Ackerman has been and still is involved in medical research and he has presented the results of his scientific research at international and national scientific meetings. Dr. Ackerman has been Medical Director of a University pain medicine department and has been Medical Director of Pain Medicine at two private hospitals. Dr. Ackerman has published over one hundred and thirty peer reviewed scientific articles and has published numerous book chapters in medical textbooks. This book is his ninth book he has published. He has been nominated previously for the Southern Medical Society Research Award as well as the Bristol-Meyers Squibb Award for Distinguished Achievement in Pain Research. He has been an expert witness in pain related medical-legal cases.

www.ingramcontent.com/pod-product-compliance
Lightning Source LLC
Chambersburg PA
CBHW020854180526
45163CB00007B/2496